C. ERGGELET ∎ B. R. MANDELBAUM

Principles of Cartilage Repair

About this Book

The subject of articular cartilage defects represents an acute clinical problem. How many people during your consulting hours, in your practice or amongst your friends complain about joint pain, combined with functional limitations or a decrease in their level of performance?

Clinical studies, recommendations and glossy product catalogues provide information and suggest solutions. Unfortunately, there is no "quick-fix method" for an instant and successful treatment of articular cartilage defects. The knowledge of orthopaedic surgeons and scientist is still fragmentary and coherence between defect morphology and pain appears to be extraordinarily complex.

Only individual treatment plans combining a well balanced choice of various options will be successful. In-depth knowledge of operative and non-operative techniques is mandatory as well as preventory strategies. What are todays possibilities, how do they work and for which patients are they successful? This book should help to answer some of those questions.

Acknowledgements

It is impossible to compose a journal article without help and input from others – and even more so a whole book. I wish to thank those who supported our project by critical questions, detailed answers, active help or patience.

Special thanks go to Dr. G. Volkert and Mrs. P. Elster at Steinkopff Publishers, who have directed my ideas onto the right track with their hearty and competent support.

The excellent graphics were realized by Mrs. R. Baumann, who also deserves special thanks.

Zürich and Santa Monica,
Spring 2008

CHRISTOPH ERGGELET
BERT R. MANDELBAUM

Contents

Introduction

Articular Cartilage Biology

Intact articular cartilage is commonly called "hyaline". Its thickness reaches 5 mm within the knee joint. Properties such as almost frictionless articulation of joint surfaces and the ability to absorb mechanical stress are owed to its unique and complex architecture.

Histologically we can differentiate between four structural zones, which differ in both composition and arrangement of its components. The thin superficial zone hosts a relatively high number of cartilage cells (chondrocytes). They stretch out into a long, oval shape parallel to the joint surface. High cell density is characteristic for this zone. In the adjacent transitional zone cell density appears to be lower with a less organized geometric arrangement of cells. The deep zone shows the lowest cell density, leaving plenty of room for cartilage matrix. The calcified zone of articular cartilage is separated from subchondral bone by the tidemark (Fig. 1). The tidemark zone is a metabolically active layer as well. Hyaline cartilage mainly consists of chondrocytes, collagens and proteoglycans as well as 80% of water.

Chondrocytes

All tissue components in articular cartilage are synthesized by chondrocytes. They make-up approximately 1% of the tissue volume. The different arrangement of cells within the tissue points towards their metabolic activity. After closure of the epiphyseal gap chondrocytes loose their mitotic activity which has a major effect on intrinsic healing capacity of articular cartilage. Degenerative cells are not replaced. Chondrocytes' endogenous ability to repair defects is limited to an alteration of synthetic performance which produces inferior cartilage matrix.

Collagen

Collagen fibrils are protein structures and resemble the largest portion of macromolecules in articular cartilage. They provide about 60% of cartilage's dry weight. The framework of hyaline cartilage predominantly consists of collagen type II and to a lesser extent of collagen types IX, X and XI. Collagen fibrils are responsible for cartilage's resilience and its ability to withstand sheer forces.

Proteoglycans

Proteoglycans consist of a core protein with chains of glycosaminoglycans connected to it. Both water uptake and output of articular cartilage are regulated by these molecules. This is particularly important for the absorption of mechanical stress as well as for cartilage nutrition since the majority of nutrition is accomplished via synovial diffusion.

Chondroitin-sulfate, Keratan-sulfate and Dermatan-sulfate are the most important representatives of all known proteoglycans.

Intact articular cartilage undergoes repetitive turnover, which is regulated by chondrocytes. Cell-matrix interactions are presumably mediated by mechanical stimulation, i.e.

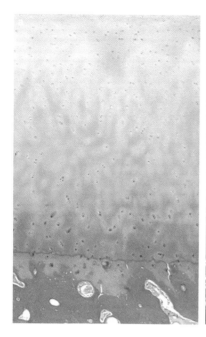

Fig. 1a, b. Histological image of human articular cartilage with HE staining (**a**) and under polarized light (**b**) (with kind permission of S. Roberts, Oswestry, UK).

through chondrocytes' short cilia reaching into the matrix. They monitor changes in mechanical loading.

This theory shows its clinical relevance for example during immobilization of a joint, which leads to rapid cartilage deterioration. Enzymatic influence through synovial diffusion is also known to affect articular cartilage. Increased synthesis if Interleukin-I promotes degradation of proteoglycans.

Articular cartilage is free of nerves, blood or lymphatic vessels. Cartilage initially receives nutrients through blood perfusion from subchondral bone during early childhood. As the calcified zone forms during skeletal maturation, flow of nutrients from subchondral bone is inhibited and cartilage becomes dependent on diffusion of nutrients from the joint cavity. Intermittent mechanical loading with consequent absorption and output of fluids plays an important role. Lack of blood supply stipulates a mostly anaerobic metabolism. Chondrocytes are capable of maintaining their metabolism even under extremely low oxygen partial pressure (less than 1% of the normal oxygen partial pressure). All glycolytic processes still function under these conditions.

During the fourth decade of life, intact articular cartilage begins a degradation process and cell-density decreases. Additional qualitative and quantitative changes of synovial fluids contribute to an early onset of tissue deterioration. Protein content and viscosity of synovial fluids in particular decrease with age.

Chondrotoxic substances (i.e. Interleukin-I) are released from the synovial membrane causing matrix degradation such as unmasking of hyaline matrix. Proteoglycans of inferior quality are released into the matrix due to altered chondrocyte synthetic activity. Initially already slow matrix turnover (approx. 800–1000 days) may thereafter cease completely.

Macroscopic changes of tissue may be depicted by changes of both colour and altered resilience. Juvenile cartilage is commonly described as being of white-blueish colour and unique taut-resilient turgor. With increasing age, hyaline cartilage appears yellow and brittle. Mechanical stiffness tested by indentation is not only decreased in areas showing surface fibrillations.

The subchondral bone plate

The subchondral bone plate resembles the tidemark between articular cartilage and subchondral bone. Although it was once assumed that cartilage nutrition is accomplished by bone marrow, we now know that this might only play a role during childhood. Moreover, resilience of the subchondral bone plate plays an important role in joint biomechanics and decreases with age. Progressing sclerosis of this thin layer is accompanied by a noticeable degeneration of the cartilage above as shown in numerous research studies. "Therapeutic" damage to the subchondral bone plate should be minimized during all treatment procedures.

Etiology of Articular Cartilage Lesions

Trauma

Isolated traumatic lesions of articular cartilage are rare. Polytraumatic injuries are frequently seen making concomitant cartilaginous lesions look far less important. Nevertheless, blunt impacts may cause chondral tears in the knee or ankle joint (Fig. 2). Traumatic patella luxations may also cause cartilage disruption. Anamnestic reports of stabbing pain with a total loss of muscle control in these cases commonly point towards a cartilage injury. Despite spontaneous reposition of the patella with only a mild joint effusion a cartilage lesion should be taken into diagnostic consideration. Conventional x-ray may only identify osteochondral fractures. However, isolated cartilage lesions may easily be identified by magnetic resonance imaging.

Fig. 2. a 3-D reconstruction of a cartilage defect on the femoral condyle. **b** 3-D reconstruction of a complex fracture of the tibial head. **c** Intraoperative picture of a traumatic grade IV cartilage lesion of the talus.

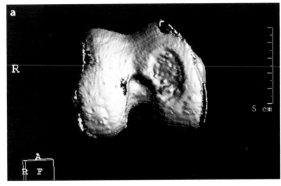

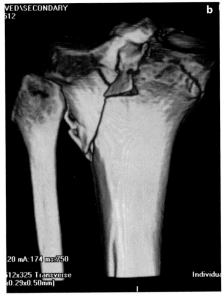

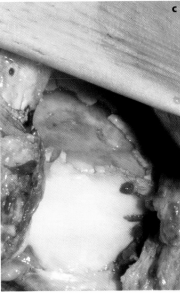

Malalignments

Axial malalignments lead to local overload in certain compartments of a joint. Cartilage degeneration and focal, compartmental osteoarthritis often follows.

Long leg standing films secure the diagnosis and are essential for planning further therapeutic steps (Fig. 3). If an axial deformity is presumed to be the main cause of a cartilage lesion, a correctional procedure should be performed prior to or at the same time as cartilage-specific therapy.

Intertrochanteric valgus or varus osteotomies may be used for axial deformities of the hip joint. Additional flexion component may be added if necessary.

Axial malalignments of the knee is often multifactorial. Changes of the condylar level or a medial or lateral sloping of the tibial plateau ought to be detected. Tibial deformities such as varus or valgus deformities must also be taken into consideration. Precise planning of the operative procedure while considering all planes is essential. For example medial deviation of the talar joint plane following successful high tibial osteotomy for example may

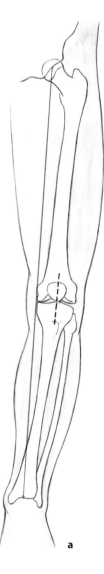
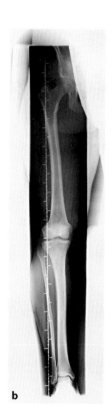
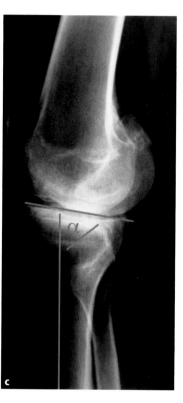

Fig. 3. a Schematic image of a varus deformity with medialization of the mechanical axis (*Mikulicz's* line). **b** Long-leg standing plain radiograph (AP view) for determination of the mechanical axis of the leg. **c** Radiograph of the knee joint (side view) with illustration of the a.p. slope of the tibia.

only avoided by precise planning of the procedure.

Two different "philosophies" exist for the different surgical techniques: open or closed wedge. Please refer for more details to the corresponding chapter.

Meniscus

The importance of intact menisci for both joint function and integrity of cartilage is undisputed. Extensive studies showed that about 90% of patients who had undergone total meniscectomy developed osteoarthritis of the affected joint compartment after 5–10 years. Even partial meniscectomy leads to cartilage deterioration in many cases – either by means of altered joint biomechanics or compartmental mechanical overload due to disturbed joint surface congruence (Fig. 4). A very careful and minimal meniscectomy is highly favourable to prevent consequent cartilage degeneration. On the other hand, partial meniscectomy of highly degenerative meniscal parts or loose tears is also important prior to cartilage-specific therapy to decrease abrasive wear.

Meniscal refixation and reconstruction should be taken into consideration especially in young patients. Defects of the medial meniscus such as tears in the pars intermedia might be bridged with collagenous meniscal implants (CMI) if the meniscus' outside rim is still intact (Fig. 5). CMI is a meniscoid, biodegradable protein-construct, which may be implanted and sutured arthroscopically (Fig. 6). Bleeding from the intact red zone of

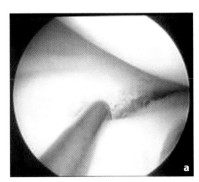

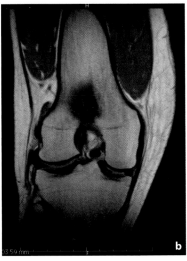

Fig. 4. a Arthroscopic view of a meniscal lesion. **b** *Bucket handle* lesion of the medial meniscus (arrow) on MRI.

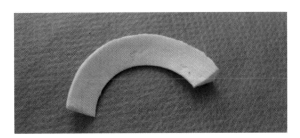

Fig. 5. Collagen meniscus implant (CMI®).

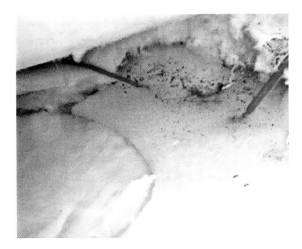

Fig. 6. Collagen meniscus implant after arthroscopic implantation in situ. Implant fixation was achieved by *inside-out* technique using non-resorbable suture.

the meniscal rim leads to formation of meniscus-like repair tissue after one year. Long term follow-ups of this procedure are not available to date. Nevertheless, operative risk of this arthroscopic procedure appears to be rather low.

▌ Distributors:
  ReGen (CMI©)

Various techniques are described for the reconstruction of missing meniscal tissue in the lateral compartment in combination with a missing intact lateral meniscal rim. However, clinically only transplantation of allografts has been proven successful (Fig. 7). Implantation may be achieved with or without bony fixation. Commonly, an arthrotomy is necessary for this procedure however recent advances in instrumentation have allowed this to become an arthroscopic procedure. Besides limited graft supply, rejection reactions and graft shrinkage are common pitfalls limiting a widespread use of the technique. Complete absence of the lateral meniscus requires allograft transplantation as the only possibility to restore joint function for a longer period of time.

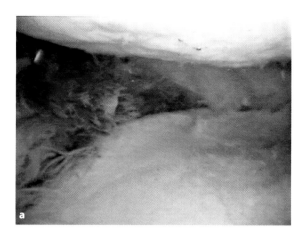

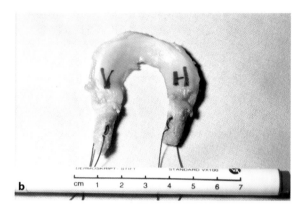

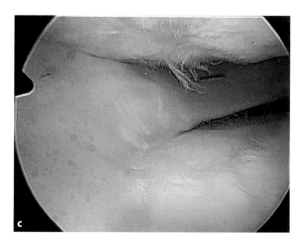

Fig. 7. a Complete loss of the lateral meniscus. **b** Human meniscus allograft prior to implantation (lateral meniscus with attached bone plug and markings for front and back). **c** Arthroscopic view of a lateral compartment in the knee 1 y after lateral meniscus allograft transplantation.

Instability

Similar to malalignments and meniscal lesions, joint instability may impair regular joint function leading to cartilage degeneration. Anterior cruciate ligament tears are of major clinical importance and need to be treated surgically concomitantly or prior to the treatment of a cartilage defect (Fig. 8). Injuries of the posterior cruciate ligament and dorso-lateral joint capsule instability are not as common but nonetheless of major importance for joint function. Further details on the various surgical techniques for the reconstruction and stabilization of knee joint ligaments shall be found in numerous references addressing these special topics.

Ligamentous instability of the ankle joint may also cause cartilage degeneration and should be treated using suitable surgical procedures.

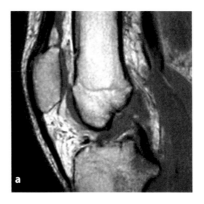

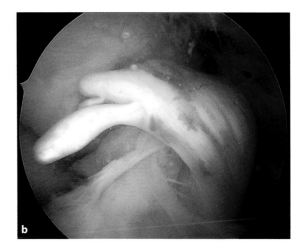

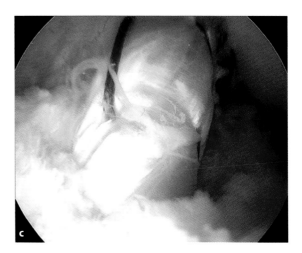

Fig. 8. a Anterior cruciate ligament (ACL) rupture on MRI. **b** Arthroscopic view of a ruptured anterior cruciate ligament. **c** Arthroscopic view of a reconstructed ACL with autologous semitendinosus transplant.

Osteochondrosis dissecans (OD)

OD often remains symptomless for many years and is often diagnosed fortuitiously by x-ray. Slow separation of osteochondral fragments from subchondral bone characterizes the disease. Segmental malperfusion, genetic predisposition and microtrauma are currently prevailed as etiologic factors. All joints of the human body might be affected but most commonly, OD is seen in the knee, elbow and ankle joint.

Definite assessment of a fragment's stability may exclusively be achieved arthroscopically (Fig. 9).

Restricted weight bearing or immobilization of the joint could be a treatment option especially in young patients with in situ fragments and open growth plates. It was recently

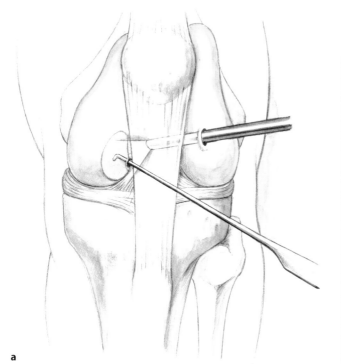

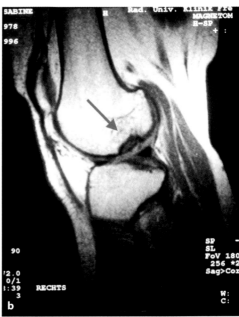

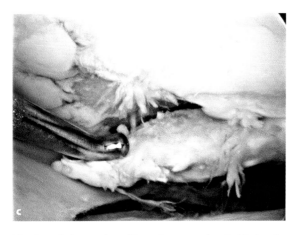

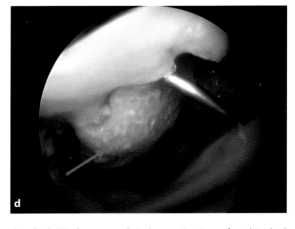

Fig. 9. a Arthroscopic probing of an osteochondral lesion for determination of its stability. **b** Osteochondritis dissecans (OD) on MRI (arrow). **c** Arthroscopic view of a partially detached OD fragment. **d** Arthroscopic view of a detached OD fragment.

reported that extracorporal shock wave therapy might be successful in the treatment of OD. However, verified data is not yet available.

Retrograde drilling has been successful in patients with persistent symptoms (Figs. 10, 11). Results from both knee and ankle joint are available to date. Anterograde drilling is not recommended as it causes further damage of the joint surface. Suitable instruments also allow performance of this procedure in the ankle and most other joints.

Retrograde bone grafting may serve as an alternative at the cost of a much more invasive procedure. The bottom of the lesion is reamed with a cannulated reamer and the bone canal filled with autogenous cancellous bone graft. Bone graft may be taken from the tibia or by turning a reamed out cylinder around ("inside-out-technique"). Advantage of this technique is that fresh spongiosa with a high healing potential is put into the lesion without damaging the cartilage surface. However, invasive nature of the procedure and

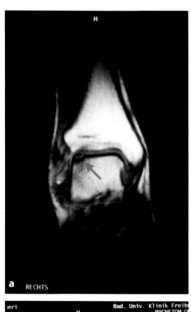

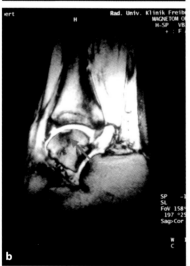

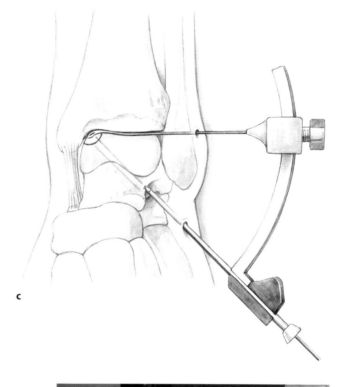

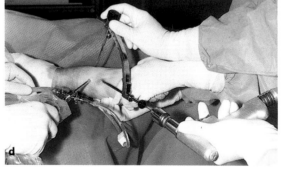

Fig. 10. a, b Talar OD lesion on MRI (coronal and sagittal plane). **c, d** Intraoperative view of retrograde drilling of an OD-lesion on the talus-shoulder using a guide instrument under arthroscopic control (**c**). Schematic procedure outline (**d**).

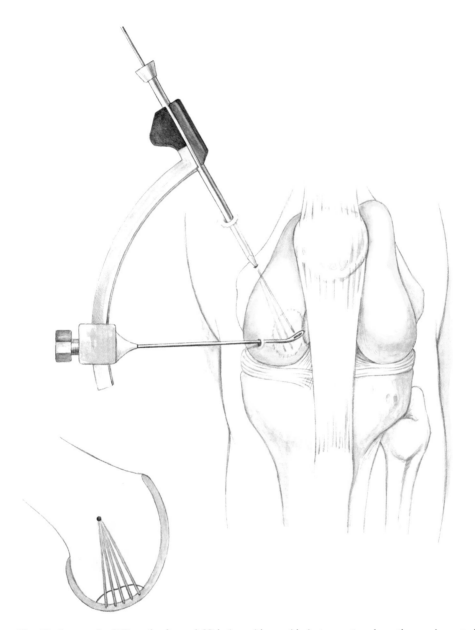

Fig. 11. Retrograde drilling of a femoral OD-lesion with a guide instrument under arthroscopic control.

risk of bleeding from the donor site are disadvantageous.

A set of cannulated reamers and instruments commonly used for osteochondral transplantations may be useful for this procedure.

OD fragments should be removed in case of partial or complete detachment. The bottom of the lesion should then be debrided and possibly filled with autologous cancellous bone graft. Larger osteochondral fragments

with a diameter greater than 1 cm may be reattached (see below). It is important to debride the base of the lesion prior to reattaching to promote a healing response. This procedure should always be considered as an attempt at repair and should be communicated as such with the patient. Alternatively, one may wait for the formation of fibrocartilage in smaller defects. Larger lesions can be covered with autologous chondrocyte transplan-

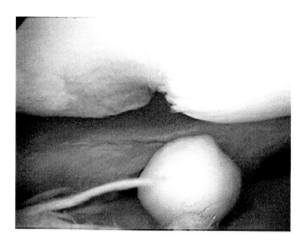

Fig. 12. Arthroscopic view of a loose body in the knee joint. Being caught between articulating surfaces it caused a track lesion on the femoral condyle.

tation after a minimum waiting period of six months, or simultaneously during a 'sandwich procedure'. Additionally, fragments may be reattached using an osteochondral plug.

A detached fragment is well likely to cause secondary damage to adjacent articular cartilage (Fig. 12).

Further details of surgical procedures are outlined below.

Osteoarthritis

Contemporary knowledge of osteoarthritis (OA) is understood to be a disease of the entire joint and not only a pathologic degradation of articular cartilage. A proposed pathomechanism suggests inflammation of the synovial membrane elicits a release of chondrotoxic proteins and leading to a progressive destruction of articular cartilage (Fig. 13). The process is furthermore accelerated by pain related functional impairment and limited perfusion. In case of general, primary OA, isolated treatment of cartilage lesions will be of minimal success. Cold weather conditions and overload due to physical exercise may cause acute, temporary exacerbation of symptoms.

Instability, meniscal lesions and malalignments have been suggested as secondary causes of OA. This symbiosis suggests an interrelationship which can be described as 'The Functional Unit' of articular cartilage. Any alteration in alignment, meniscus or ligamentous status is intimately linked to the integrity of articular cartilage. Successful treatment of those may stop or at least decelerate cartilage degeneration. Treatment of focal degenerative cartilage lesions may follow in a second-step procedure, as outlined in this book.

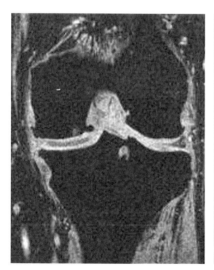
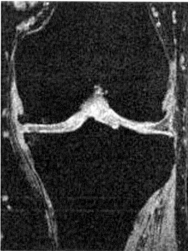
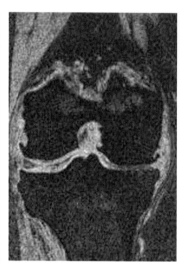

Fig. 13. a MRI-image of the knee joint, presenting progressive articular cartilage degeneration (from left to right) (coronal view, T1-weighted 3D FLASH water excitation) (with kind permission of C. Glaser, Munich, Germany).

Rheumatoid arthritis

Polyarthric strike and progressive joint erosion are characteristic for this sytemic disease. However, etiology remains undetermined. Immunologic processes are assumed to be part of its pathogenesis. Some other diseases from the variety of rheumatoid disorders (psoriasis, *Reiter's* syndrome, Lupus erythematosus and many more) may be accompanied by a monoarthritic or polyarthritic symptom complex. In these cases extensive diagnostics are essential to exclude a chronic, specific inflammatory process responsible for joint pain.

This is also true for reactive or post-infectious arthritis. If at all, they may only be diagnosed by direct or indirect detection of bacteria, i.e. yersinia, chlamydia, borrellia, streptococcus or their specific toxins.

Interdisciplinary therapeutic approaches are to be favoured over mostly frustrating attempts to solely restore articular cartilage. Symptomatic therapies like lavage, debridement or synovectomy, however, are often appropriate to improve function and ease pain.

Genetic factors

Most genetic disorders are of multifocal nature. Familiar increase of chondromalacia-like cartilage lesions combined with ligamentary laxity could have its origin in genetic alteration of collagen synthesis. Further diagnostic steps should be taken in these cases in collaboration with a center of hereditary disorders. Therapeutic options still remain the same. However, the outcome is likely to be less successful if the basic disease remains untreated.

Obesity

Overweight and obesity are proven risk factors for the development of osteoarthritic erosions of articular cartilage. Combination with post-traumatic conditions increases likelihood of OA development to 80%. Importance of weight control for both prevention and therapy of articular cartilage lesions has to be part of planning a dedicated therapy. Weight loss may prevent joint function impairment, lengthy drug intake and risky surgical procedures. Therefore, collaboration of dieticians, physiotherapists and even special hospitals are desirable. Surgical intervention for the treatment of severe cases of obesity may even be an alternative.

Interactions between a particular diet or so called "balanced" nutrition concepts in shape of tablets, capsules or fluids and certain osteoarthritic lesions have not been depicted yet. Nevertheless, it remains unquestionable that a well balanced diet is beneficial for all tissues and structures of the human body.

Cartilage tumors

Most benign and malign tumors of chondral origin located close to joints are to be characterized radiographically by certain unique patterns and distinct structures of bone and cartilage. Amongst those, giant cell tumor, chondromyxoid fibroma, osteochondroma, periosteal chondrome and enchondroma ought to be mentioned. Diagnosis of the rare chondroblastoma is more difficult. It is usually accompanied by cartilage destruction and is localized in the periphery of the knee joint and in the humerus. Mainly children and adolescents are affected. A round, immediate subchondral osteolytic cyst is often found. Cyst may also penetrate into the joint cavity.

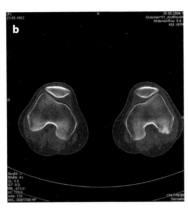 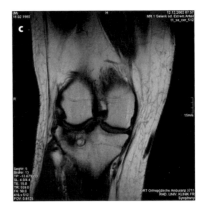

Fig. 13. b CT scan of a chondroblastoma of the distal femur with arrosion of the cartilage (with kind permission of G. Herget, Freiburg, Germany). **c** Enchondroma of the distal femur with cartilage arrosion on MRI (with kind permission of G. Herget, Freiburg, Germany).

Plain radiographs sometimes show some scattered mineralizations within the cyst. Prognosis after curettage is good. Following complete cure, larger defects should be scheduled for cartilage reconstruction.

Microtrauma

Even minor damage of articular cartilage such as repeated microtrauma may lead to degenerative changes in cartilage matrix. Loss of proteoglycans and appearance of atypical collagens type I, III and X can be observed. Chondrocytes may degenerate or show focal proliferation. Intrinsic changes cannot be identified from outside. They will eventually lead to accelerated cartilage degeneration with loss of its biologic stability. Current imaging techniques may only identify progressed stages of disease.

Superficial erosions of articular cartilage stimulate surrounding chondrocytes to temporary increase their metabolic and mitotic activity. Increased proteoglycan and collagen type II levels can be identified within the juxtacellular matrix. However, this process is not capable of restoring the lesion.

Deeper lesions, such as osteochondral defects, usually heal like all other inflammatory processes. However, subchondral bone must be exposed to allow release of mesenchymal stem cells into the defect. These cells still have the ability to differentiate into cartilage- and bone-producing cells such as chondrocytes and osteoblasts. Like formation of scar tissue of the skin, osteochondral defects will be filled with fibrous repair tissue. Compared to hyaline cartilage, it shows inferior metabolic and biomechanical properties. Fibrocartilage is not capable of bearing mechanical loads of the main weight bearing areas and will degenerate over time.

Diagnostics

Clinical examination

Cartilage defects are unlikely to be diagnosed by clinical examination. Solely hemarthrosis or locking symptoms may suggest existence of a traumatic osteochondral lesion. Presenting symptoms are usually increased overall knee pain following strenuous physical activity. Pain is commonly not to be localized by triggering classic pressure points.

Use of one or several scoring systems with different main foci are recommended to be used in standardized clinical examination. This is especially important in regards of future quality management in the medical field.

Clinical outcome and joint function scores exist for all joints. They describe a joint's function at any time point during therapy. Examples of different scoring systems are described in the appendix of this book. Use of these scoring systems is highly encouraged.

Radiography

Cartilage defects cannot be identified by plain radiographs. Joint space narrowing or intensified subchondral sclerosis may at most suggest existence of chondral lesions. OD lesions can only be identified in later stages of the disease.

Nevertheless, routine diagnostics require plain radiographs in at least two different views (AP and lateral) (Fig. 14). Omitting those, one might oversee etiologically important pathology of the bone. Importance of radiographic imaging in determination of mechanical axis has been emphasized in one of the former chapters. Weight bearing views are vital to demonstrate joint space narrowing that may not be present if the joint is not loaded. The addition of postero-anterior flexion views increase the sensitivity to evaluate joint space narrowing (Rosenberg).

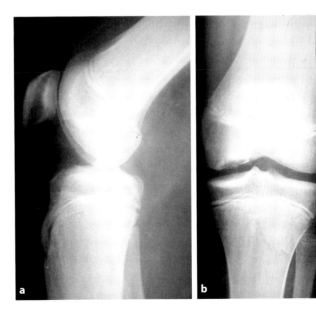

Fig. 14 a, b. Plain radiographs of a knee joint with osteochondritis dissecans on the medial femoral condyle. Lateral view (**a**), AP view (**b**).

Magnetic resonance tomography

Magnetic resonance tomography (MRT, also referred to as "magnetic resonance imaging", MRI) plays a major role in diagnostics of articular cartilage defects. This non-invasive technique offers the possibility to evaluate not only cartilage surfaces but also thickness of articular cartilage (Fig. 15).

The modified, descriptive Outerbridge-Classification is widely accepted:

0 Normal cartilage
1 Superficial fibrillations
2 Cartilage lesion reaching max. 50% of cartilage thickness (erosion)
3 Cartilage lesion reaching 50–100% of cartilage thickness (ulceration)
4 Subchondral bone exposed.

Additionally, cartilage volume and concomitant intraarticular lesions may be identified (joint effusion, synovitis, ligamentous or meniscal injuries).

Definition criteria and guidelines for standard MRI examinations and additional examinations or protocols for special demands are not available to date (Fig. 16).

T1-weighted spin echo sequences produce precise anatomic images of both subchondral bone and cartilage.

Discrimination between synovial fluid and cartilage surface is achieved by T2-weighted images. This technique shows a sensitivity of up to 90% and a specificity of up to 96% for the identification of degenerative cartilage lesions. Cartilage lesion diagnostics using MRI techniques were revolutionized by the introduction of T1-weighted, fat-suppressed, 3D-gradient echo sequences. Fat-suppression techniques decrease disturbing bright signals from adjacent fat of subchondral bone. 3D data acquisition produces slice thicknesses with a minimum of 0.5–1 mm combined with infinite slice direction. Fine-tuning of certain parameters in spoiled gradient-echo techniques (i.e.

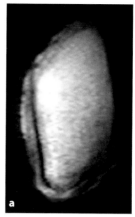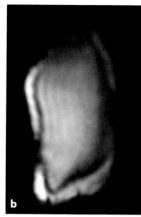

Fig. 15 a, b. MRI images of isolated patellae with Outerbridge grade I cartilage defect (**a,** T2 SE sagittal) and grade IV defect (**b,** Turbo-GE) (in collaboration with M. Uhl and T. Bley, Freiburg, Germany).

FLASH, Fig. 17 a) allows intensifying signals of articular cartilage for better contrast to surrounding tissues and synovial fluids.

Still, identification of histochemical or ultrastructural changes in articular cartilage by MRI is in its nascent stages. Intraarticular or i.v. injections of negatively charged ionic contrast-enhancement molecules hours prior to the examination combined with joint exercise are currently used in some centers to assess biochemical properties of articular cartilage (Fig. 17 b).

MRI follow-up examinations for clinical purposes should always be performed on the same magnetome for better comparability of images.

The following MRI sequences are recommended standard protocols used for articular cartilage imaging:

T1-weighted spin echo sequence (SE)
T2-weighted turbo spin echo sequence with fat suppression (TSE)
T1-weighted fat suppressed gradient echo sequence with 3D data acquisition, short echo time
TE (for example 10 ms), short repetition time TR (for example 50 ms) and with a small to moderate flip angle (30°).

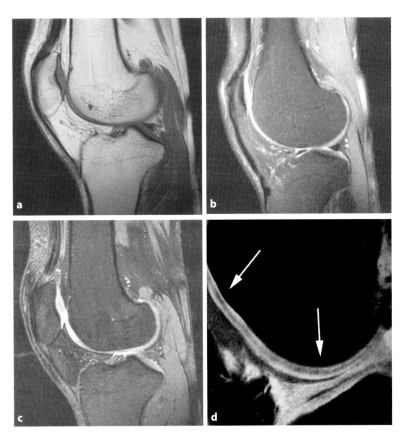

Fig. 16a–c. MRI images of the knee, sagittal slices: **a** T1-weighted spin echo sequence (SE), **b** T2-weighted turbo spin echo sequence with fat-suppression (TSE) and **c** T1-weighted, fat-suppressed gradient echo sequence with 3D data acquisition (in collaboration with M. Uhl, Freiburg, Germany).

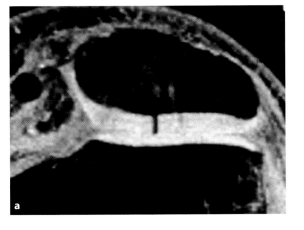

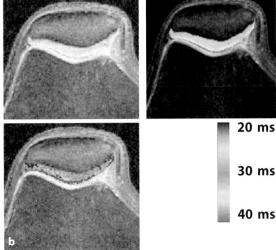

20 ms

30 ms

40 ms

Fig. 17. a MRI image three months after pin fixation of a patellar osteochondral fracture following traumatic patella dislocation. T1-weighted 3D FLASH water excitation sequence with i.v. gadolinium enhancement.

b MRI image with quantitative mapping of transverse relaxation time (T2-time) of cartilage: typical increase of T2-time from deep zone to superficial zone (with kind permission of C. Glaser, Munich).

Joint imaging is usually performed in coronary and sagittal slices. Only special demands require additional sequences such as STIR-sequences for evaluation of subchondral bone edema. Availability of all slices in print and digital form is desirable and advantageous for diagnostics and preoperative planning. Despite easier handling, MRI "snapshots" are usually non-satisfying.

Classification of articular cartilage lesions and criteria for choosing appropriate therapy

Different classifications for standardized description of cartilage lesions are currently in use. The Outerbridge scale is most commonly used (Fig. 18):

Grade 0:	Intact articular cartilage
Grade 1:	Cartilage softening, intact joint surface, focal colour change
Grade 2:	Superficial fissuring
Grade 3:	Fissures and fragmentation extending into the matrix
Grade 4:	Erosion reaching the subchondral bone plate. Eburnated bone.

Experienced surgeons often use the ICRS score for more subtle tasks (International Cartilage Repair Society score/see appendix).

Generally speaking, determination and evaluation of the following cartilage defect characteristics is necessary to choose the appropriate cartilage repair technique.

Localization

Defect localization plays an important role, especially with regards to potential surgical treatment. Lesions located away from the main weight-bearing area of a joint, such as on the far posterior femoral condyle, might not require immediate surgical treatment. Anterior knee pain in retropatellar cartilage injuries may be multifactorial and often persists even after successful cartilage therapy. Morbidity of the surgical approach has to be taken into consideration under certain circumstances, i.e. in surgical treatment of OD lesions on the dorsal shoulder of the talus or the femoral head. Furthermore, single lesions are usually easier to treat than multifocal lesions.

Concomitant injuries

Untreated concomitant injuries (instability, meniscal injuries, and axial malalignments) often limit potential success of cartilage defect therapy. The joint works as a functional unit where any change in one factor can affect the others via *Chondral Overload Syndrome (COS)*. The excess load via malalignment, obesity, meniscal or ligament deficiency leads to cartilage break down, and ultimately defects in different stages:

▌ Stage 1: Pain from subchondral bone overload
▌ Stage 2: Fissures
▌ Stage 3: Articular cartilage defects

Defect size/Containment

Defect sizes ought to be measured as exactly as possible. Defect sizes correlate closely with the degree of containment and tribologic intactness of the joint (Fig. 19 a–d). The following measures are determined for the human knee:

Defects smaller than 2 cm^2 are usually surrounded by stable cartilage shoulders and are

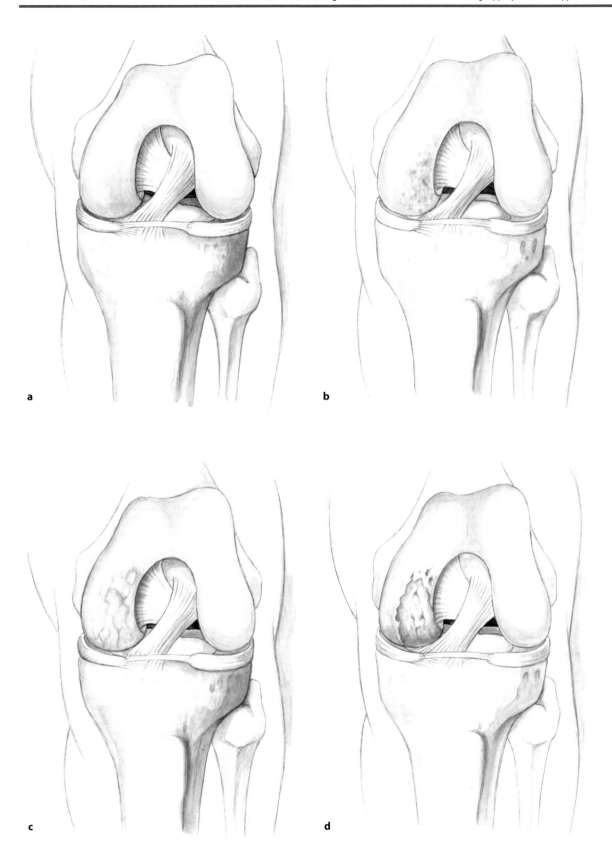

Fig. 18. Cartilage defects grade I–IV according to the Outerbridge scale (**a–d**).

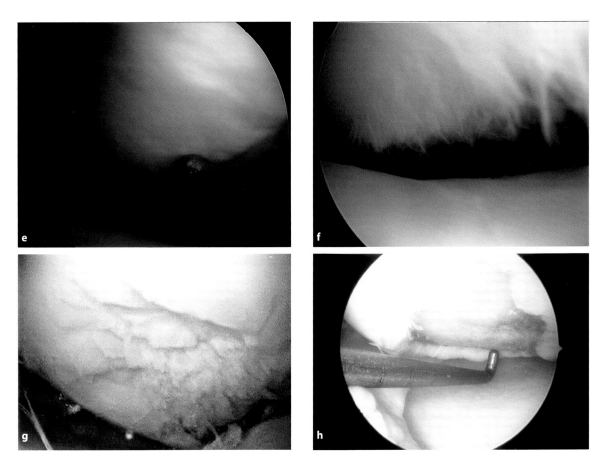

Fig. 18. e Arthroscopic view of a cartilage lesion Outerbridge grade I with colour change to yellow and softening of the surface. **f** Arthroscopic view of a cartilage lesion Outerbridge grade II with superficial fibrillations. **g** Arthroscopic view of a cartilage lesion Outerbridge grade III with substantial ulcerations of the cartilage. **h** Arthroscopic view of a cartilage lesion Outerbridge grade IV – the subchondral bone is visible.

therefore well protected from further mechanical loading. Up to a size of 5 cm^2, containment will be preserved. However, mechanical stress on surrounding cartilage will be critically increased causing continued degenerative processes. Defects larger than 5 cm^2 with destroyed containment show direct contact of eburnated bone with the corresponding articular surface, causing rapid destruction of the whole compartment. Joint space narrowing can be identified on plain radiographs. Size definitions may vary depending on the patient's bodily constitution. This may affect therapy recommendations based on defect size. Measuring round or elliptical defects may be particularly difficult and results are often inaccurate (note: ellipse area = A × B × 3.14) (Fig. 19 e).

If 3D-reconstructions of diseased joint compartments are not available, determination of defect volume and size has to be done arthroscopically. Graduation on commonly used probe hooks has been proven to lack accuracy. Intraarticular structures are often described larger than they really are. A graduated needle may be useful instead. It may easily be inserted into the joint from various positions parallel to the defect margins. Dedicated graduation allows accurate measurements (Fig. 20).

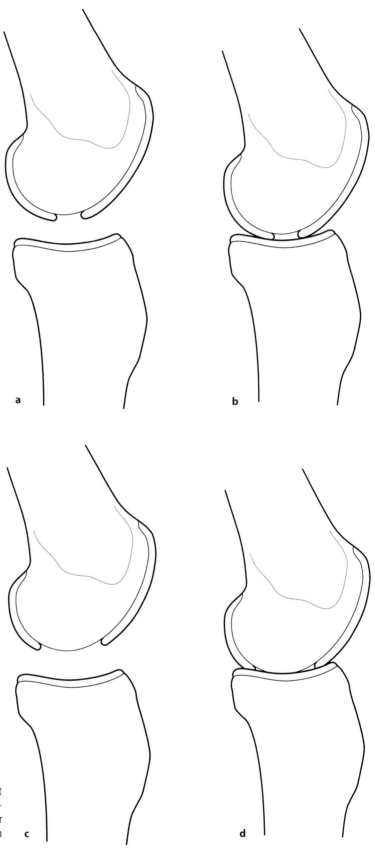

Fig. 19a–d. Small cartilage lesions do not interfere with correct articulation of joint surfaces (containment) (**a, b**). However, larger lesions grossly interfere with the articulation of joint surfaces (**c, d**).

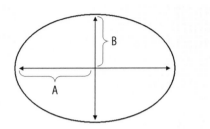

Fig. 19 e. Surface calculation of an ellipse ($A \times B \times \pi$).

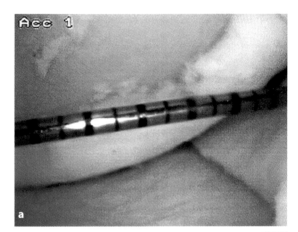

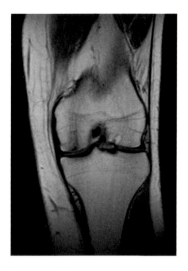

Fig. 21. MRI image of the knee (coronal) with identification of subchondral cysts on the femoral condyle.

Radiography/MRI

Subchondral cysts (Fig. 21), focal bone necrosis or tumors have to be excluded as potential etiologic factors of a cartilage lesion.

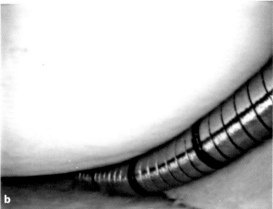

Fig. 20 a, b. Arthroscopic identification of a cartilage defect on the femoral condyle. A graduated canula (**a**) or a flexible wire (**b**) is inserted for exact determination of defect size.

Conservative Treatment

Conservative Treatment of Articular Cartilage Defects

Drug treatment

Innumerable drug preparations are available for the treatment of articular cartilage lesions. Ongoing research studies show effectiveness. According to recommendations of leading specialists' associations, all drugs besides NSAIDs and pure analgesics are divided into two groups: "Slow acting drugs in osteoarthritis" (SADOA) and "disease modifying osteoarthritis drugs" (DMOAD).

All currently clinically available "cartilage drugs" belong to the group of symptomatically acting drugs ("symptomatic slow acting drugs in osteoarthritis" – SYSADOA). Some early results suggest that some preparations may have a positive influence on cartilage morphology and may decelerate or even halt the process of progressive cartilage destruction. Still, it is extremely difficult to find proof for both pharmacologic potential and the quality of their effects. Lack of objective biochemical, immunologic and simply descriptive parameters for quality control is apparent.

Until the use of OA modifying drugs is established for the treatment of cartilage lesions, one has to focus on symptomatic improvement of both pain and joint function.

Use of so called "alternative" substances (herbal drugs, homoeopathic preparations) as a base therapy over a period of 3–6 months may help to reduce intake of NSAIDs, which are known for various severe side effects.

A list of substances – not claiming completeness – commonly used for treatment of articular cartilage lesions is printed below.

To date, no clinical research studies exist proving that certain drugs have the potential to inhibit development of cartilage degeneration, decelerate or reverse degenerative processes. Nevertheless, several drug preparations are claimed to successfully treat cartilage defects or cartilage degeneration. According to different models of efficacy various substance groups are to be defined.

Non-steroidal anti-inflammatory drugs (NSAID)

NSAIDs show rapid effect onset but only short-term efficacy. They show both analgesic as well as anti-inflammatory effect by inhibition of prostaglandin synthesis. First generation substances of the NSAID-group in particular have severe side effects. About one third of all clinically treated gastric ulcers and one third of all fatalities due to gastric ulcers account for intake of NSAIDs. Still, prophylactic combination of NSAIDs with gastric protective drugs (for example PPIs – *proton pump inhibitors*) is disputable not only for economic reasons. Use of second and third generation drugs may reduce risk of gastro-intestinal side effects by approximately 50%. Drug efficacy results from inhibition of cyclooxygenase-2 (COX-2). To date, extensive comparative studies with non-selective NSAIDs are pending.

▎ Short-term efficacy
Mephenamine, Diclofenac, Dexibuprofen, Naproxene, Ketoprofene, Ibuprofen, Salicylic acid.

∎ **Medium-term efficacy**

Proglumetacine, Lonazolac, Acemetacine, Indometacine.

∎ **Long-term efficacy**

Meloxicam, Lornoxicam, Piroxicam. Pyrazolones also show long term effects but ought to be used restrictively due to risk of accumulation and overdosing especially in the elderly.

∎ **Gastric protection drugs**

Antacida

H2-receptor inhibitors:

Cimetidine, Ranitidine, Famitidine.

∎ **COX-2 inhibiting NSAIDs:**

Coxibes.

Neuroceuticals

∎ **Glucosamines.** Chondroitin-sulfate is one of the main components of hyaline cartilage. Both proteoglycan deficiency and chondroitine sulfate deficiency have been shown in osteoarthritic cartilage as well as in degenerative cartilage of different etiology. It remains controversial whether or not insufficient uptake of cartilage-specific nutrients in the gastrointestinal tract plays a role in deficiency. Chondroitines are widely available as nutrition supplements especially in English speaking countries. However, resorption rates of the gastrointestinal tract are known to be rather low with the recommended TID dosing but recent clinical data has shown that, when taken all at once, serum levels are high. Medication with glucosamines has not yet shown to be effective in OA for cartilage regeneration. However, it is assumed to have prophylactic efficacy by means of replenishing structural deficiencies. Analgesic as well as anti-inflammatory effects from regular oral medication with glucosamines are uncontentious. Different research studies have proven such and were conducted according to requirements of up-to-date evidence based medicine.

Green lipped mussel and shark cartilage extracts are offered for therapy of OA and other inflammatory processes due to their high contents of glucosamine sulfate and glucopolysaccharides. Bioavailability of active ingredients from these extracts, however, is considerably lower than in preparations containing pure glucosamine sulfate. Additionally, biologic extracts often contain pollutants – not to mention ethical concerns in obtaining shark cartilage. *In vitro* investigations have shown that supplementation of human chondrocyte cultures with glucosamines enhances proteoglycan synthesis. Daily oral intake of 1500 mg of glucosamine sulfate is currently recommended.

Flavonoids as well as Avocado and Soy oil have shown efficacy in clinical and preclinical studies but are less common for clinical use.

∎ **Stinging nettle.** Stinging nettle has been used in folk medicine as tea or fresh juice to treat rheumatic and osteoarthritic symptoms for ages. 13-HOTrE is nowadays believed to be the active ingredient and has also been isolated as such. This ingredient inhibits chondrotoxic cytokines, namely TNS-a and Interleukin-1. Macrophages are known to synthesize these substances and release them as a reaction to joint inflammation. Both TNS-a and Interleukin-1 promote synthesis of cartilage destructing enzymes and enhance further release of inflammatory mediators such as prostaglandin.

Besides anti-inflammatory and minor analgesic effects stinging nettle extracts and their active ingredients may also have prophylactic effects on joint destruction. Daily oral intake of 8–12 g of active ingredient is recommended.

∎ **Devil's claw.** Devil's claw originates from South Africa and is also commonly used in folk medicine. Various preparations of the herb's tuber-shaped roots were used to treat fevers, tumors, skin lesions and also for pain relief. Its main active ingredient is believed to be *Harpagosit*. However, its mode of efficacy remains unknown. Anti-inflammatory and analgesic effects seen in clinical application are partially explained by influencing the arachidonic acid metabolism. Recommended daily intake is approximately 30 g of *Harpagosit*. Various clinical studies could show pain relief as well as anti-inflammatory effects in many cases.

▮ **Willow.** Extracts from willow bark contain flavonoids and *salicin*. Ancient scripts of folk medicine as well as placebo-controlled studies report anti-inflammatory and analgesic effects. A maximum of 120 mg salicin are recommended as daily oral intake. Exact modes of efficacy for the drug remain cryptic. Due to its content of salicylates use should be restricted in patients under Marcumar therapy. However, platelet function does not seem to be affected.

▮ **Enzymes.** Enzymes function both as initiators and inhibitors of inflammatory reactions in the human body. Various enzyme "cocktails" are currently available to inhibit inflammatory joint disease. Application may occur orally or intra-articularly. Modes of efficacy remain – once more – cryptic. Clinical studies reported effects such as pain relief in patients with OA of the knee. Due to various different active ingredients of commercially available preparations recommendations for daily oral intakes cannot be made.

▮ **Interleukin antagonists.** Interleukins play an important role in modulating inflammatory processes of our joints. Interleukin 1-*a* in particular initiates synovitis when applied in high dosage and may also break down articular cartilage through various chains of reaction. Small cartilage defects and other joint pathologies may initiate increased release of interleukins. High Interleukin-1 concentrations may be compensated to a certain degree by monocytically synthesized Interleukin-1-receptor antagonists. However, chronic pathologies may not be compensated by this mechanism.

Interleukin receptor inhibition is initiated via external administration of high dosages of Interleukin receptor antagonists into a diseased joint. Such Interleukin receptor antagonists are recovered autologously from the patient's blood. Six ampoules of highly concen-trated, autologous Interleukin-1 receptor antagonists are available after three weeks. According to preliminary clinical studies, pain relief and improved joint function may be achieved up to three months post injection.

It remains to be proven if or to which extent this therapy may actually improve cartilage morphology or decelerate cartilage degeneration. According to the manufacturer the method is currently not recommended for patients with late stage OA.

▮ **Cortisone.** Intra-articular administration of cortisone for the treatment of acute inflammatory joint processes is widely used. However, efficacy is induced indirectly through a positive influence upon improved cartilage nutrition by instant pain relief. The decreased pain therefore improves joint mobility. The long-term effects of cortisone administration have been shown to degrade articular cartilage. Therefore, long-term therapy with intra-articular injections of cortisone is not indicated.

▮ **Hyaluronic acid.** Hyaluronic acid (more precisely: Hyaluronan) is a key molecule in synovial joints. Hyaluronan deficiency or alteration of its biomechanical characteristics, due to inflammatory processes or OA, leads to functional impairment and increased joint surface friction. Hyaluronan is synthesized by both chondrocytes and cells within the synovial membrane. Hyaluronan and proteoglycans serve as water absorbers within articular cartilage and therefore catalyze indirectly nutrient diffusion into the matrix. Endogenous hyaluronan is responsible for viscosity of synovial fluids. These fluids cover the entire joint surface and also fill the joint cavity. Additional protection of the joint surface from toxic mediators is currently being discussed.

Hyaluronan undergoes changes in quality and quantity in response to cartilage lesions or to OA. Viscosupplementation with exogenous hyaluronan was developed to improve functional impairment seen in degenerative or injured joints. This therapy is supplementary which provides symptomatic effects. Numerous studies suggest a preventive component of the therapy, as the progress of cartilage degeneration is decelerated by protection of the joint surface. However, cartilage regeneration has not yet been observed.

Generally speaking, all joints may be treated with exogenous hyaluronan. However, one has to take into consideration that not all drug preparations are approved for all joints. Molecular weight of macromolecules also differs, whereas one should prefer medium molecular weights as they most closely match physiologic conditions.

Preparations differ in production mode for hyaluronan. Both fermentative production and extraction from tissue – mostly from animals – is used. Best results are achieved in patients with mild to moderate degenerative changes seen on radiographs. Besides well known risks of intra-articular injections, effusions and reversible swellings of the joint may rarely be observed. Allergenic potential of animal proteins and inaccurate injection technique are assumed to be the cause. Hyaluronan therapy is not indicated in rheumatoid, gouty and infectious arthritis. Serial weekly injections are recommended, depending on the commercial product used. Interestingly, some patients have reported so-called "carry-over-effect", expressing low pain or pain-free periods of time after treatment periods of several months.

Viscosupplementation with hyaluronan may relief pain and improve joint function in many cases.

▌ **Gene therapy.** Gene therapy focuses on altering various key cells in the joint. Distinct alterations of cells' genotype shall preferably be achieved in a long-lasting manner.

Stimulation of monocytes for continuous synthesis of increased amounts of Interleukin-1-antagonists or implantation of genetically altered chondrocytes continuously synthesizing mature cartilage matrix is conceivable. Different laboratory techniques may transfer new genetic information on cell populations by "bombardment" with DNA-fragments or through transfection of cell populations with viruses as carriers of genetic information.

Therapeutic potential of those techniques appears to be almost unlimited for the entire field of medicine, not only for cartilage therapy. Nevertheless, responsible handling of such techniques and knowledge as well as effective ethical control is indispensable.

Clinical applications of gene therapy approaches are not yet available.

Physical therapy

Various physicotherapeutic interventions for treatment of cartilage injuries are used. They focus on relief of pain and improvement of joint function. Regeneration of injured cartilage is not to be expected. Nevertheless, progressive degenerative processes may be decelerated serving as active OA prophylaxis. By improving muscle tone and restoring joint motion, a shock-absorber effect is seen decreasing pain and force across the joint.

Physical therapy is mainly used in conservative therapeutic approaches or if surgical procedures are not yet indicated. It might also be used preoperatively to improve certain motion patterns to accelerate healing processes postoperatively.

Physiotherapy

In the case of intra-articular lesions, pain will lead to reactive functional impairment of the affected joint. Painful movements will not be performed anymore leading to shrinkage of the joint capsule and consecutively to a decrease of blood perfusion.

In order to break this vicious circle, physiotherapy uses different techniques and focuses on the following goals:
▌ Pain relief by lowering weight-bearing (positioning, traction, walking aids)
▌ Manual stretching of painful, contract joint capsules (possibly by means of physical measures)
▌ Detonisation of hypertonic, periarticular muscle groups and passive mobilisation of the joint

▪ Improvement of joint mobility by active, active-assisted and passive mobilisation of joints

▪ Improvement of muscular joint stabilization by well-directed treatment of muscular deficiencies

▪ Improvement of joint function by learning compensatory techniques and coordinative exercises

▪ Medical training therapy for improvement of locomotive qualities (power, motion economy, endurance, coordination).

Progressive joint degeneration following cartilage injury can only be decelerated or prevented by maintaining physiologic motion patterns. Knowledge and research in the field of joint physiology cannot be covered exhaustively within this book.

Bandages and orthosis for the treatment of gonarthrosis

Besides medication, surgical therapy and physiotherapy, concomitant treatment with bandages and orthotic auxiliaries is indicated in many cases of gonarthrosis. However, the main disease will not be controlled by these means. Nevertheless, it might be possible to ease pain and improve joint function.

▪ **Bandages.** Bandages are easy to use which is especially important for the elderly. Stocking-like stretch-material can easily be slipped on and gives patients a feeling of stabilization. This impression originates from tissue compression by elastic material. True support will not be achieved with these bandages.

Another effect of OA bandages seems to be temperature control. Many elderly patients report exacerbation of pain in cold and humid weather conditions. This may be reliably prevented by using bandages.

Proprioceptive qualities of bandages are accepted nowadays, however, there is no detailed proof for this phenomenon. Nevertheless, it is beyond doubt that bandages may improve muscular activity patterns around injured joints by means of their propriocep-

tive quality, as reported in several clinical studies. Influences on both effusion- and co-ordination-mechanism shall be mentioned here.

Inwoven fabric pads allow administration of gentle pressure upon certain joint compartments. This is of particular interest in case of retropatellar cartilage lesions. Various bandages allow improved patella tracking and may therefore biomechanically unload osteoarthritic joint facets. Pain relief may be achieved in many cases.

▪ **Orthosis.** Orthosis are characterized by a combination of stable support apparatus' and bandage components for the treatment of diseased joints. Above described effects may therefore be achieved using these devices.

Additional qualities come into effect in orthosis-therapy. Rigid support apparatus' allow external joint stabilization to a certain extent. Patients with late stage OA, showing completely degenerated knee joints with instability may regain the ability to walk. Dedicated hinges allow (un-)limited motion and support joint function. In addition, flexion limitation may be useful following surgical procedures or in case of retropatellar OA.

Use of knee joint orthosis' is especially important in conservative treatment of medial or lateral gonarthrosis. Unicompartmental osteoarthritic changes are often accompanied by varus deformations following medial meniscus lesions or medial meniscectomy. In general, these cases need surgical axial realignment. However, performance of a surgical procedure may not be feasible due to various reasons. Orthosis-therapy may then offer the opportunity to administer valgus or varus stress to unload affected joint compartments (Fig. 22).

Postoperative use of so-called "OA-splints" following meniscal reconstruction or cartilage repair techniques has also been proven to be useful. Preoperatively, they may convince patients in need of a valgisation tibial osteotomy of the usefulness of the procedure by simulating expected outcomes.

Different studies could show compartmental unloading of specially designed OA-orthosis'.

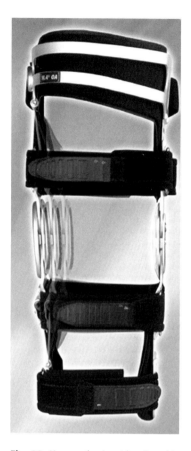

Fig. 22. Knee orthosis with adjustable varus/valgus stress.

In summary, orthosis' and bandages are useful auxiliaries in the treatment of gonarthrosis, capable of easing pain and improving joint function. In certain cases, compartmental unloading by OA-orthosis' may decelerate disease progress. However, causal therapeutic approach cannot be achieved.

Electrotherapy

Electrical currents may alter both mitotic and synthetic behaviour of human cells. The spectrum of effects reaches from pain relief by affection of pain-conducting nerve fibres to destruction of genetic material.

Electrotherapy focuses on application of defined current-qualities to accomplish certain effects.

The following chapter introduces the most important techniques:

- low frequency currents (< 1000 Hz)
- Stanger's bath
- Iontophoresis: transcutaneous ion transport for increased uptake of positively or negatively charged drug containing gels.
- Transcutaneous Electrical Nerve Stimulation (TENS): solely symptomatic local pain relief by means of blockage of pain transmission. Application of mostly square pulse currents is achieved through battery-driven pocket devices.
- Medium-frequency currents (1000–300,000 Hz)
- High-frequency currents (> 300,000 Hz).

Currents are applied without direct skin contact but produce local heat effects by electromagnetic waves by means of chemical reactions within the skin (diathermy). This specific therapy offers the advantage of reduced cardiovascular stress compared to exogenous heat application.

Pulsed signal therapy

Pulsed signal therapy (PST) is currently advertised as to restore articular cartilage. This therapeutic goal shall be achieved by application of defined square pulse, low frequency direct current. It could be shown experimentally that chondrocytes' ability to proliferate is positively influenced by application of electrical currents in general and PST's unique pulse pattern in particular. Additionally, chondrocytes' synthetic performance shall be enhanced by improved water absorption of injured cartilage. Clinical studies could show both improvement of pain symptoms and joint function. However, morphologic changes of injured articular cartilage by application of PST could not be shown, yet. Studies did not meet common standards and expectations of evidence based medicine. Significant side-effects of this therapy have not been reported. Therapy costs are currently not carried by national health insurances.

Ultrasound

Ultrasound therapy for treatment of diseases of the locomotive system has been widely used for many years. High-frequency currents ranging from 800 Hz and higher are used. These currents are converted into mechanical vibrations by means of quartz and are then forwarded onto the body. Vibrations may achieve temperature increase, especially in layers between different tissues. This may lead to improved blood perfusion, metabolism and nutrition. Direct effects onto articular cartilage has not yet been shown,. However, different studies could show indirect chondroprotection by means of buffering inflammation mediators released from activated synovial membranes. Formation of fibrocartilage in osteochondral defects with penetration of the subchondral bone plate could be stimulated by application of ultrasound. Reviewing the Cochrane Library one comes to the conclusion that there is no evidence-based efficacy for therapeutic use of ultrasound in gonarthrosis therapy.

Magnetic fields

Although there are reports from folk medicine that magnetic fields are beneficial for diseased joints, contemporary medicine foresees no indication for using low intensity magnetic fields in joint therapy. Pulsed magnetic field therapy is currently intensively promoted for the treatment of sports injuries and OA. Therefore, advocates of this therapy also believe in possible treatment of articular cartilage defects. Increased energy supply within tissue shall be achieved by means of pulse modulation of magnetic waves which then shall increase oxygen partial pressure within the tissue of interest. Beneficial effects of these processes for bradytrophic tissues such as articular cartilage and meniscus are stressed in particular. Liu et al have conducted a study in 1996 to investigate effects of pulsed magnetic field therapy on extracellular matrix of articular cartilage. However, the majority of research studies in this field focuses on osteoneogenesis. Side-effects of this therapy have not yet been reported.

Costs for application of pulsed magnetic field therapy are currently not carried by national health insurances.

Extracorporeal shock wave therapy

Extracorporeal shock wave therapy (ESWT) has been used for the destruction of kidney concrements for many years. After development of smaller devices and improved focus technology, ESWT has been introduced into clinical orthopaedics throughout the last decade. High and low energetic impulses are used for treatment of calcific tendinitis, lateral epicondylitis as well as heel spurs. Treatments with low energy devices can be performed without analgesia and additional radiographic control in most cases. Penetration depth of impulses reaches around 35 mm.

Low penetration depth makes ESWT not suitable for the treatment of articular cartilage defects. However, high energy devices may be useful for treatment of OD lesions in which the sclerotic zone in the depth of the lesion could be penetrated by means of high

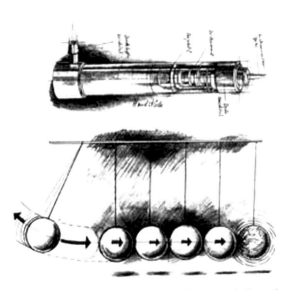

Fig. 23. Contemporary image showing the mode of effect of extracorporeal shock wave therapy (with kind permission of EMS, Konstanz, Germany).

energy impulses. With intact cartilage surface on top of the fragment reintegration seems possible. Results of this new application have not yet been published. It also remains to be proven whether or not pain in retropatellar chondromalacia may be positively influenced by ESWT. Possible side-effects of ESWT include temporary exacerbation of symptoms and superficial skin irritations.

Cost coverage of ESWT by national health insurances is still being discussed controversially.

Operative Treatment

Operative Treatment of Articular Cartilage Defects

In contrast to conservative therapies, operative interventions are capable of covering a cartilage defect completely – by transplantation and regeneration of tissue or by refixation of detached fragments.

Refixation of detached cartilage fragments

In case of acutely and traumatically detached osteochondral fragments one should always attempt to reattach it in anatomically correct position. Newly detached OD fragments may be reattached with high success rate, especially in young patients.

▍ **Principle.** Anatomically correct refixation of (osteo-)chondral fragments with resorbable pins, screws, fibrin glue or by means of osteochondral plugs.

▍ **Surgical procedure.** Arthroscopic inspection easily detects the previously diagnosed defect. However, traumatic defects may limit arthroscopic overview considerably by bleeding from subchondral bone. It may still be apparent days after acute injury. Large fragments are usually easily put into place correctly. Smaller fragments often have to be transferred from joint recesses back to its correct anatomic site. Sometimes smaller fragments are still attached by small tissue bridges. If the traumatic episode occurred greater than 1 week prior to surgery, removal of fibrous tissue from the depth of the defect might be necessary. Blood clots which may look like fibrous tissue at times shall not be removed.

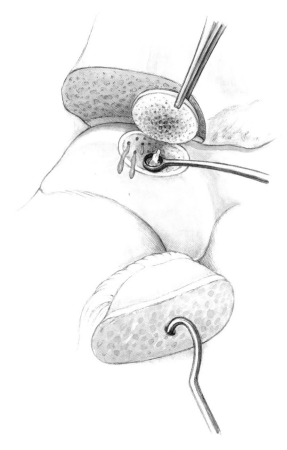

Fig. 24. Debridement of a cartilage lesion on the talus shoulder after retracting a partially detached osteochondral fragment prior to refixation (approach via a medial malleolar osteotomy).

Partially detached OD fragments are to be considered as special cases. In these mostly young patients refixation attempts should always be undertaken. This does not apply for solely chondral fragments with a diameter < 1 cm. However, every successful refixation is preceded by debridement and penetration of mostly sclerotic fragment beds (I have a great arthroscopic picture if you need this for example with K-wires >1.6 mm) (Fig. 24).

For treating shoulder, elbow or hip joints it is usually necessary to use an arthrotomy. Medial malleolar osteotomy usually provides sufficient exposure of the ankle.

Fixation with resorbable pins

Two pins shall at least be inserted into the fragment and the underlying subchondral bone with use of special instruments (Figs. 25, 26). It is especially important not to align pins parallel to each other in order to achieve more stable fixation. Increased stability is achieved with cannulated pins (smart nails$^©$).

▌ Advantages
– Resorbable material
– Arthroscopic technique
– Only thin perforation of fragment.

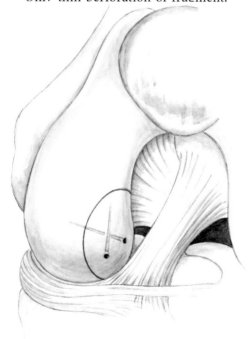

Fig. 25. Fixation of an osteochondral fragment on the femoral condyle using resorbable pins.

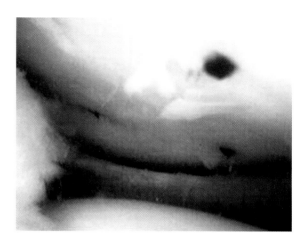

Fig. 26. Arthroscopic view after fixation of an osteochondral fragment using resorbable pins (Ethicon).

▌ Disadvantages
– Insufficient compression of fragment to bone possible
– Fixation less stable compared to screws.

Fixation of osteochondral fragments with screws

After reposition, detached fragments may be fixed with small fragment spongiosa (cancellous is the term we use in America) screws. For oval defects one screw may be sufficient as rotation is unlikely to occur. Alternatively one may use resorbable screws. Reoperation is necessary after healing to remove the hardware.

▌ Surgical procedure
– Insertion of a K-wire which matches small fragment cannulated screw system
– Pre-drilling using cannulated drill bits guided by K-wires
– Insertion of screw and tightening
– Levelling of the screw's head with surrounding cartilage.

Specially designed instruments are available from manufacturers of resorbable screws.

▌ Advantages
– Stable fragment fixation
– Arthroscopic technique.

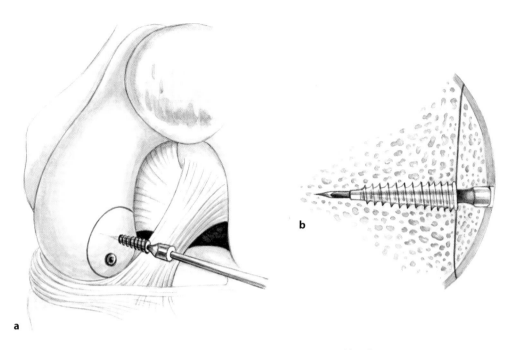

Fig. 27 a, b. Fixation of an osteochondral fragment by inserting cannulated screws over a guide-wire.

❚ **Disadvantages**
- Damaging of corresponding joint surface by prominent screw's head
- Comparably large drill canal (troublesome with smaller fragments)
- Necessity of material removal when using metal screws
- Formation of osteolysis possible when using resorbable screws.

Fragment fixation with fibrin glue

In case of refixation of small fragments in areas outside the main weight bearing area using open technique, fibrin glue fixation may be sufficient. However, stability will be less compared to other techniques. Temporary immobilization of the joint may be necessary.

❚ Supplier:
Tissucol Duo (Baxter Bioscience).

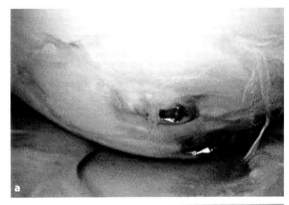

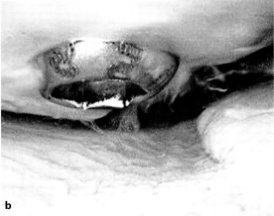

Fig. 28 a, b. Arthroscopic image after fixation of an osteochondral fragment with screws (**a**). Note the track lesion caused by the screw-head on the articulating surface of the tibia (**b**).

Fragment fixation with osteochondral plugs

Fragments are fixed with autologous osteochondral plugs using press-fit technique (Fig. 29). For this procedure one may use standard instruments sets commonly used for osteochondral transfers.

▮ Surgical procedure
- Plugs are removed from the lateral aspect of the trochlea or from the intercondylar notch (it might be necessary to use plugs from the ipsilateral knee joint when treating other joints)
  Important: often recommended "standard length" of osteochondral plugs of 1.2 cm is not sufficient. They should be at least 2 cm in length. Diameter of plugs should be no less than 4 mm, preferably 6 mm
- Drilling of recipient hole of matching size through the fragment into the subchondral bone, according to dimensions of instruments
- Insertion of osteochondral plug while paying attention to surface congruity.

▮ Advantages
- Autologous fixation, no artificial material
- Arthroscopic technique
- Reconstruction of the fragment's cartilage surface.

▮ Disadvantages
- Large drill canal (fracture risk!)
- Low compression of fragment onto subchondral bone.

Postoperative treatment

Postoperative treatment may vary, depending on the type of surgical procedure performed and stability of chosen fixation methods. Joint unloading for approximately six weeks is recommended. Follow-up examination including plain radiographs is often not successful and MR-imaging often impossible due to artefacts caused by metal implants.

Non resorbable screws ought to be removed after 6–8 weeks as they may lesion the corresponding joint surface.

Refixation of purely chondral fragments is usually less successful but should still be considered, especially in young patients. Penetration of unclosed growth plates in young patients with large diameter and/or long implants must be avoided.

Patients are to be informed that these procedures are considered to be attempts to preserve autologous tissue and therefore secondary procedures for the removal of re-detached fragments may be necessary.

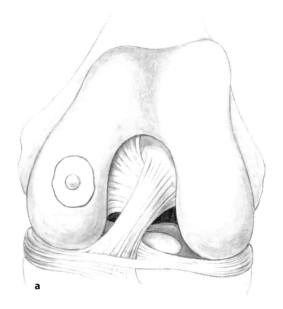

a

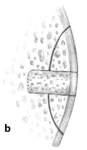

b

Fig. 29 a, b. Repair of an osteochondral defect on the femoral condyle using an autologous osteochondral plug.

Medial malleolar osteotomy

Cartilage defects of the ankle joint may force the surgeon to perform a medial malleolar osteotomy for achieving sufficient exposure of posterior defects in case an anteromedial approach (ventral wedge technique) is not successful (Fig. 30).

▌ Surgical procedure

– Forward-curved skin incision across the medial malleolus
– Determination of osteotomy level using a K-wire under control of image intensifier
– Placement of possibly two partially threaded spongiosa screws (cannulated, if necessary to be guided by K-wires) under image intensifier control. Screws shall not be fully inserted. Threads of the distally inserted screws must be placed completely proximally from the planned osteotomy level

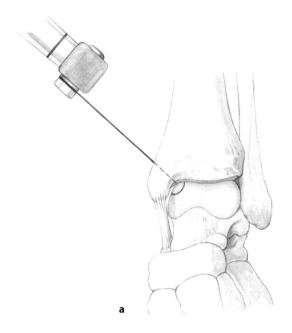

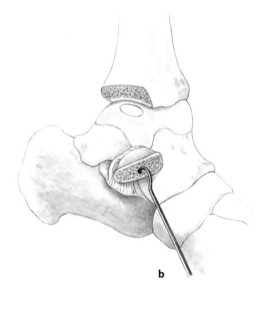

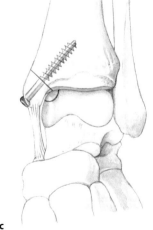

Fig. 30 a–c. Medial malleolar osteotomy for the identification of cartilage defects of the talus from medially. **a** Axis- and angle-dependent osteotomy of the medial malleolus, **b** retracting the distal portion and **c** refixation of the malleolus after treatment with screws.

– Osteotomy of the medial malleolus with an oscillating saw. A ventrally, above the talus' edge inserted retractor or else will protect the talus from saw lesions
– Downward retraction of the medial malleolus with a single hook for sufficient joint exposure and satisfying overview
– Reposition must occur anatomically correct to avoid secondary joint injury. This is likely to be achieved when pre-drilled holes are used
– Tightening of the screws, followed by radiographic control. In case of soft bone, use of washers may be helpful

K-wires in combination with tension band fixation can alternatively be used in case there is not enough space to place two screws. This will be sufficient for rotational control. A single screw is therefore not sufficient.

Joint lavage/cartilage shaving/débridement

Performance of arthroscopic joint revision by lavage in case of substantial articular cartilage injury often leads to significant pain relief. Detached cartilage components like collagen fibrils and proteoglycans act as inflammatory mediators, causing and maintaining chronic synovitis. Removal of fragments therefore explains efficacy of joint lavage. This solely symptomatic approach will not show long lasting success. However, repetitive arthroscopic lavages may be indicated.

▌ **Indications.** Degenerative cartilage defects (in case causal therapy is not possible or not appreciated by patient).

▌ **Surgical procedure**
– Thorough lavage of the entire joint cavity with several litres of lavage fluids. Posterior joint compartments may be reached by transligamentary approach

– Cartilage shaving shall be restricted to careful removal of superficial, loose cartilage layers using a shaver
– Value of superficial cartilage treatment procedures using laser or other high-energy sources are not proven to be superior and therefore questionable.

▌ **Advantages**
– Arthroscopic technique
– Low effort.

▌ **Disadvantages**
– Temporary effect
– Symptomatic therapy.

Bone marrow stimulation techniques (drilling, abrasion, microfracture)

After anecdotal mentioning of subchondral drilling for the treatment of cartilage lesions by Pridie 1959, L. Johnson – among others – studied the principle of bone marrow stimulation scientifically. Despite inconsistent clinical results, this technique has ever since been improved and used to date for example by Steadman.

▌ **Principle.** Exposure of subchondral bone marrow allows slight bleeding into the cartilage defect site, thus initiating formation of fibrocartilaginous repair tissue (fibrocartilage) (Fig. 31). Different growth factors and enzymes are thought to be responsible for initiating this process.

▌ **Surgical procedure (arthroscopy)**
– Removal of loose and damaged cartilage with curettes until healthy tissue is exposed. *Retrograde* instruments are helpful in preparing defect edges facing towards the portal of the arthroscope
– Preparation of a stable defect shoulder.

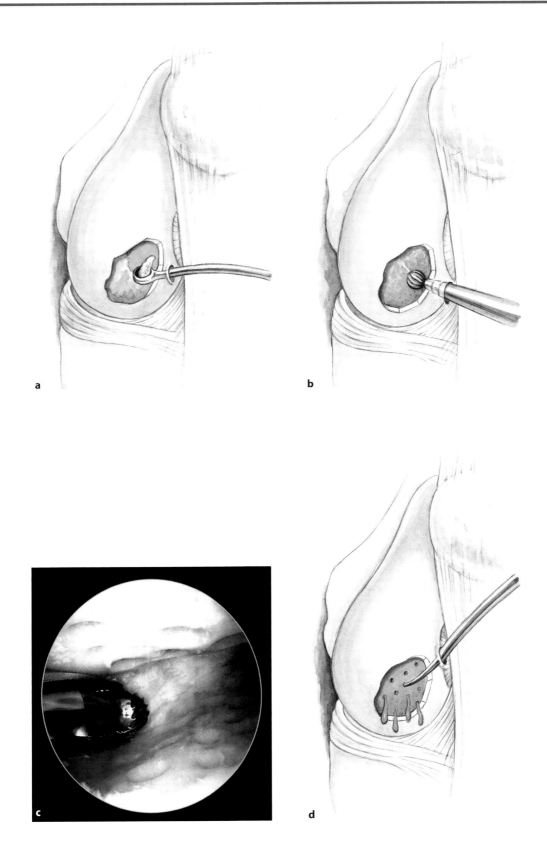

Fig. 31a–d. Bone marrow stimulation techniques: **a** cartilage defect debridement, **b** abrasion chondroplasty with a ball-shaped burr, **c** arthroscopic image of abrasion chondroplasty on the femoral condyle, **d** microfracture.

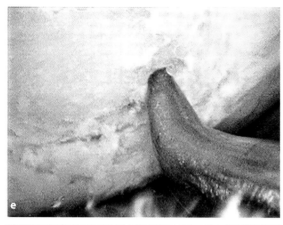

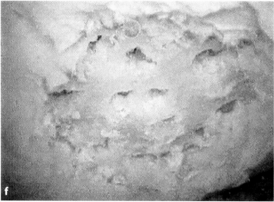

Fig. 31 e, f. Arthroscopic views of microfracture technique on the femoral condyle.

Different techniques are used:

▮ **Abrasion arthroplasty.** Exposure of subchondral bone is achieved by removing superficial bone with a shaver or better, a barrel/ball-shaped burr or acromionizer. It is especially important to include peripheral areas of the defect and avoid tapering the defect shoulder. Large, degenerative defects have to be deepened in order to achieve sufficient regenerate thickness.

▮ **Microfracture.** Perforation of subchondral bone with angled picks ("chondropick") is achieved by well-dosed mallet-blows. Sets of instruments with various angled picks (range from 0°–90°) are available from different manufacturers. Perforation of subchondral bone should be performed perpendicularly to the surface so that holes are not shaped ovally and bone bridges between holes are not destroyed. Holes should be 3–4 mm apart from each other, with a depth of approx. 4–5 mm. Some instruments are graduated. To stimulate fibrocartilage formation up to the very edges of the defect, it is particularly important to create perforations close to the defect shoulder.

Fig. 32 a, b. Anterograde drilling of an OD-lesion by penetrating the fragment on the femoral condyle (**a** front view, **b** sectioned lateral view).

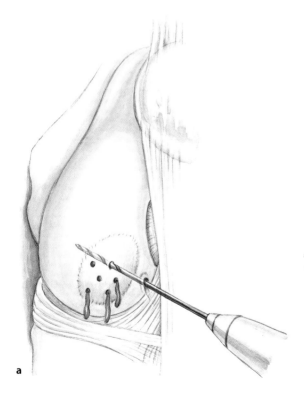

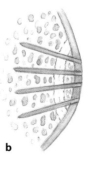

▪ **Drilling.** Above recommendations are also applicable for antegrade drilling. K-wires or small drill bits with a diameter of 1.5–2 mm are to be used to perforate the subchondral bone plate (Fig. 32).

OD lesions are special cases requiring retrograde drilling. Given an intact cartilage surface but visible demarcation of the fragment (yellowish colour, soft spot), the underlying sclerotic bone has to be perforated with a drill bit. Special guide instruments (for example from the ACL-reconstruction set) or image intensifiers are used to perform retrograde drilling without injuring overlying cartilage. Refrain from antegrade drilling through the fragment to avoid additional cartilage injury.

Heat-related necrosis and accidental injury of overlying cartilage are remaining problems of this particular technique.

▪ **Control of bleeding.** Releasing tourniquet pressure will allow moderate bleeding into the defect as well as blood clot formation (Fig. 33). If this cannot be observed, perforation/abrasion has to be repeated.

▪ **Pitfalls**
- Fracture of subchondral bone plate by overly dense or non-perpendicular perforations

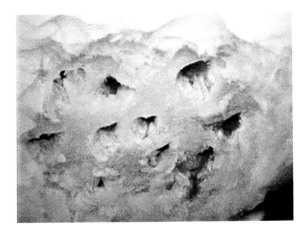

Fig. 33. Arthroscopic view of a cartilage lesion on the femoral condyle after microfracture and reduction of water/tourniquet pressure to allow bleeding.

- Incomplete defect filling because of wide gaps between perforations.

▪ **Postoperative treatment**
- Unrestricted CPM (exclusion: lesions of the femoropatellar joint; apply flexion restriction of $60°$ for 2–6 weeks in these cases).
- Unloading of the affected joint for 4–6 weeks
- Gait training with weight-bearing limitation ("soul contact" only) after procedures of knee and ankle joint.

It may take up to one year until fibrocartilage formation is completed. Hence, revision surgery is usually not indicated within a postoperative period of at least one year.

▪ **Indications**
- Full-thickness cartilage defects of all joints
- Maximum defect size varies with overall body size
- Stable defect shoulder and intact joint containment are necessary, as early regenerates are usually soft and need protection by healthy surrounding cartilage.

▪ **Advantages**
- Arthroscopic technique
- Cost efficient.

▪ **Disadvantages**
- Fibrocartilage formation only with chance of deterioration over time
- Injury of the subchondral bone plate.

▪ **Results**
- Arthroscopic: Regenerates appear to be soft with fibrillated surface even under ideal circumstances within the first 12 months. In case of a missing stable defect shoulder regenerates are likely to be torn off, resulting in failure of the procedure
- Macroscopic: Even complete defect filling with stable, smooth fibrocartilage does not necessarily result in success of the procedure. Reasons for this phenomenon are unknown.

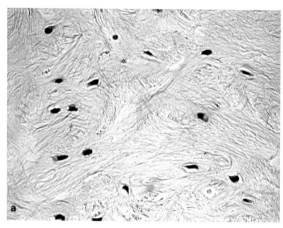
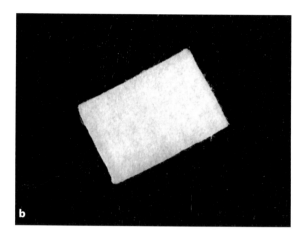
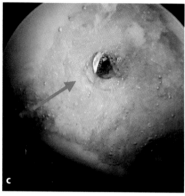

Fig. 34. a Histological image of fibrocartilage following microfracture treatment (for comparison to healthy hyaline cartilage see Fig. 1). **b** Polymer/hyaluronan fleece (Chondrotissue©) for scaffold augmented microfracture (SAMIC). **c** Arthroscopic view of a polymer/hyaluronan fleece (Chondrotissue©) for scaffold augmented microfracture (SAMIC) after fixation with resorbable pin (smart-nail©) (with kind permission of W. Petersen, Münster, Germany).

– Histological: Histological processing of regenerates shows characteristic fibrocartilaginous structure (Fig. 34) even under ideal conditions, differing significantly from hyaline cartilage.

A 3D porous and resorbable matrix for the treatment of smaller cartilage defects in combination with microfracture called Chondrotissue© demonstrated better and histologically superior coverage of the defect site in preclinical studies. The scaffold is augmented with autologous serum in a one stage procedure and fixated intraosseously with vicryl or pins.

Augmented microfracture techniques

In order to enhance cartilage regeneration after microfracture and stabilize the defect site resorbable scaffolds are used to cover a cartilage lesion after penetration of the subchondral space.

The AMIC® technique (Autologous Matrix Induced Chondrogenesis) uses a collagen membrane which is sutured to the perifocal cartilage. That way the lesion is well protected but animal studies have shown no benefit in comparison to microfracture alone.

Osteochondral transplantation

Transplantation of articular cartilage in shape of osteochondral plugs has been proven to be useful both experimentally and clinically. One has to differentiate between autologous and allogenic transplants. The availability of osteochondral allografts might be problematic in some countries.

Use of autografts in cartilage repair and its results have long since been described.

Modern sets of instruments with thin-walled core cutters allow gentle acquisition of cylindrical osteochondral transplants ("plugs"). This allows transfer of cartilage autografts in standardized sizes into marginally smaller holes within the defect for *press-fit* fixation. Harvest areas for osteochondral donor plugs are located in areas of lesser weight-bearing and also in the contralateral knee joint. Development of advanced arthroscopic techniques made osteochondral transplantations widely accepted and used.

▌ **Principle.** Transplantation of osteochondral plugs from joint compartments of lesser weight-bearing into cartilage defects for the reconstruction of an intact cartilage surface (Fig. 35).

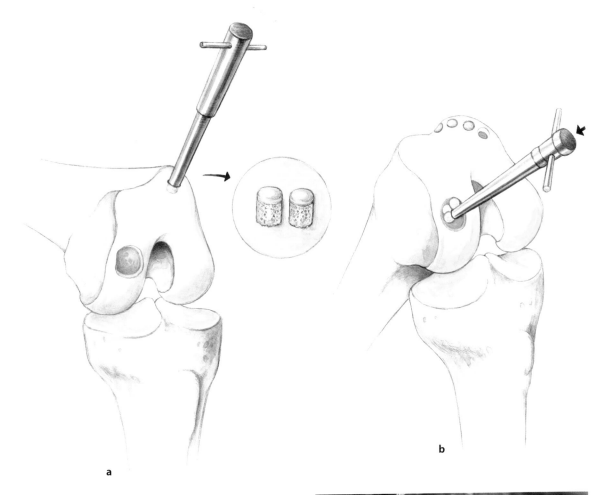

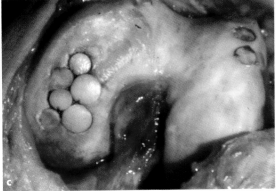

Fig. 35 a–c. Treatment of a cartilage defect on the femoral condyle using osteochondral plugs. **a** Debridement of the defect and harvesting of osteochondral plugs from areas of lesser weight-bearing. **b** Implantation of osteochondral plugs into the defect. **c** Defect on the femoral condyle after implantation of osteochondral plugs. Plugs overlap to achieve better defect coverage.

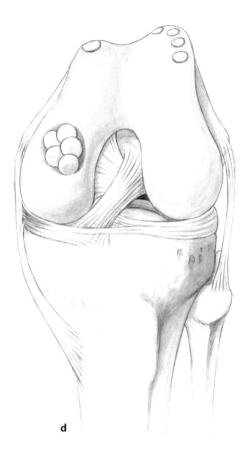

d

Fig. 35 d. Intraoperative image of a cartilage defect on the femoral condyle after implantation of osteochondral plugs.

▮ Surgical procedure

– Exposure of the cartilage defect, debridement if necessary and determination of exact defect measures. Single-use trial cylinders allow determination of needed number and size of plugs for a complete coverage of the defect.
  Note: Not all available instrument sets allow arthroscopic use!
– Arthroscopic transfer of more than three plugs should remain within hands of highly specialized and well-trained orthopaedic surgeons.
– Donor plugs are harvested according to the measured size of the defect. Core cutters are usually marked as *donor.* Preferable donor sites are medial and lateral margins of the trochlea and a smaller margin around the intercondylar notch. It is of special importance to insert core cutters perpendicu-

larly to the cartilage surface. Bone bridges between two harvest sites shall not be smaller than 3 mm to maintain stability.
Diamond cutters are available alternatively to standard stainless steel core cutters. Depending on instrument sets, recipient sites will be cut out, milled down or chiselled. Instruments are usually marked as *recipient.* Again, harvesting should be performed perpendicularly to the joint surface.
Note: It has been proven to be useful to insert plugs one by one. Plugs are to be inserted by gently pushing them out of the core cutter with a small mallet or operating a threaded mechanism. Then gently push plugs into the recipient site with using a small pestle until joint surfaces level is reached. This procedure may be repeated several times with different plug diameters until defect is completely covered.
– Harvest sites may be retrofilled with plugs from recipient sites. Thorough lavage and flexioning of the joint is followed by a final control of secure plug insertion.

▮ Postoperative treatment.
Passive motion therapy immediately after surgery with unlimited range of motion (exception: flexion limitation in case of retropatellar and trochlear cartilage lesions), limited weight bearing for 6 weeks.

▮ Pitfalls

– **Problem 1:**
  Donor plug is too long with incongruent cartilage surfaces
– **Solution 1:**
  Do not force plugs in as this usually injures the cartilage surface. Deepen the recipient site carefully with a small burr (Fig. 36 a, b)

– **Problem 2:**
  Donor plug is inserted too deep
– **Solution 2:**
  Do not let the plug "float" within the recipient site, but back the bottom with spongiosa harvested from a donor site (Fig. 36 c, d)

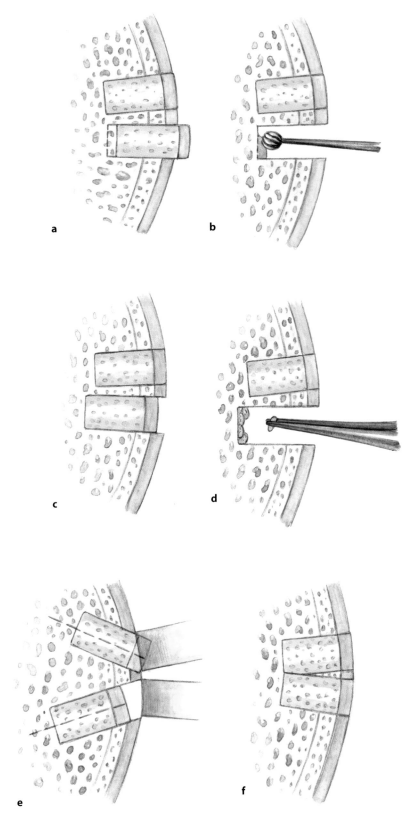

Fig. 36a–f. Pitfalls of implantation of osteochondral plugs (for explanation see text).

– **Problem 3:**
  Rotation of the plug does not match (in case of non-orthograde plug or recipient site)
– **Solution 3:**
  Prior to final impaction try to achieve best alignment using two cannulae (Fig. 36 e, f).

Note:
Defect covering cannot exceed 70%, even with closely inserted plugs. Defect cover may be improved by harvesting donor plugs in an overlapping manner or by microfracturing the small spaces between plugs (Fig. 37).

Removal of incorrectly inserted plugs without destroying them is very difficult. "Mini-cork-screws" are available for this purpose but tend to be torn out of the plug.

The so called "Mosaicplasty-System" with many small core cutters of diameters ranging from 4 to 8 mm is frequently recommended. The "Mega-OATS-System" achieves defect coverage by implanting a single plug with a diameter of 12 to 16 mm. This technique offers the advantage of improved defect coverage but bears the disadvantage of producing joint surface incongruity due to grossly different convexity of surfaces. The natural history of a Mega-OATS donor site is similar to that of an articular cartilage defect of the same size and therefore is recommended under special circumstances or when allograft is used.

Positioning, potential displacement or necrosis of transplants may be made identified by MRI. Osseous alterations and oedemas may be seen for a prolonged time in MRI-images. However, clinical outcome might still be positive (Figs. 39, 41).

Osteochondral transplantations have also been proven to be successful in other joints. Cartilage defects in shoulder, elbow, and femoral head may be covered if enough donor material is available. It might be necessary to harvest donor plugs from the knee joint. Plugs may also be harvested from to front margin of the talus (Fig. 40).

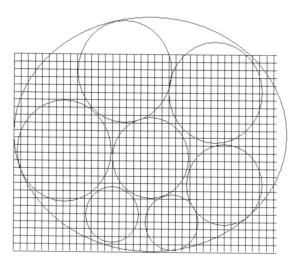

Fig. 37. Schematic image of an elliptic cartilage defect: even very tight implantation of plugs may only reach incomplete defect coverage.

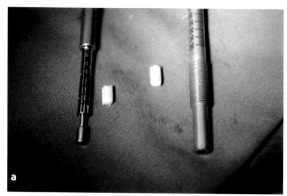

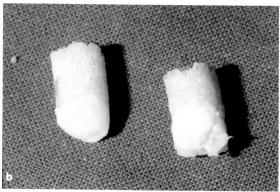

Fig. 38. a Core cutter (cannulated, round chisel) set for harvest and implantation of osteochondral plugs (Aesculap). **b** Osteochondral plugs after explantation from a defect (with injured cartilage, right) and prior to implantation (with intact cartilage, left).

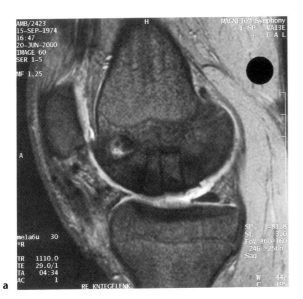

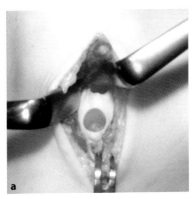

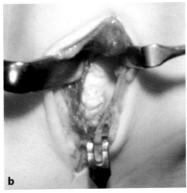

Fig. 40 a, b. Intraoperative view of the treatment of a cartilage defect on the talus' shoulder with osteochondral plugs. Ventral approach without medial malleolar osteotomy. **a** Harvesting of both recipient (top) and donor plug (bottom) with intact articular cartilage. **b** Implantation of donor plug into the lesioned weight-bearing area (top) and filling of the harvest site with the plug from the recipient site to minimize subchondral bleeding (bottom).

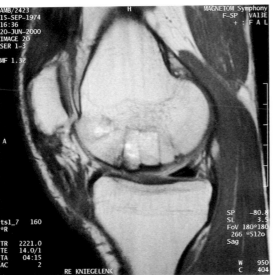

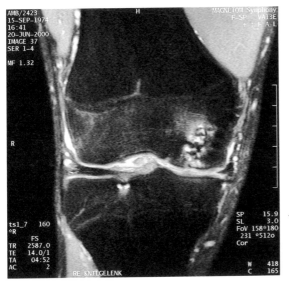

◄ **Fig. 39 a–c.** MRI of the knee with a cartilage lesion on the femoral condyle after treatment with osteochondral plugs. **a, b** Osteochondral plugs can easily be identified. Subchondral bone plate appears irregular. **c** Development of a subchondral bone necrosis.

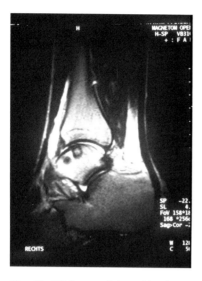

Fig. 41. MRI image of the ankle after implantation of osteochondral plugs for the treatment of a cartilage defect on the talus.

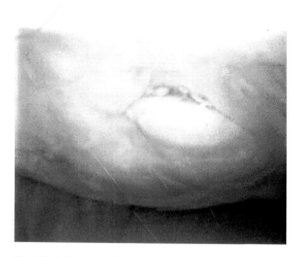

Fig. 42. Arthroscopic view 10 months after treatment of cartilage lesion on the femoral condyle with an osteochondral plug.

▮ Advantages

– Autologous tissue, no artificial materials used
– Comparably cost-effective procedure (*cave:* several sets of instruments contain single-use articles)
– Arthroscopic technique may be used with restrictions
– Transplantation of hyaline articular cartilage.

▮ Disadvantages

– Incomplete coverage of the defect
– Morbidity of donor site
– Limited availability of donor plugs
– Potential necrosis of centrally placed plugs
– Lesioning of the subchondral bone plate
– Irregular cartilage surface (Fig. 42).

To fill donor sites after osteochondral transplantation various materials have been used with no obvious advantage in comparison to empty donor sites. The morbidity of harvesting healthy cartilage from the trochlea is proven as well as the incomplete bonding between transplant and perifocal cartilage.

For retrofill and potentially for primary filling of osteochondral defects a resorbable biphasic polymer/calcium sulfate device was developed (TruFit©) as an *off the shelf* solution. Cylinders with a diameter from 5–11 mm actively incorporate spongious blood and elements to restore osteochondral defects. Preclinical studies showed next to complete osseous restoration the regeneration of a cartilage phase with a high content of collagen II. Specifically shaped implants will be available for treatment of patella/tibia or ankle lesions.

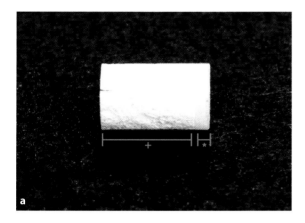

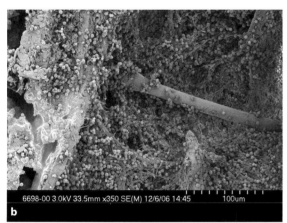

6698-00 3.0kV 33.5mm x350 SE(M) 12/6/06 14:45   100um

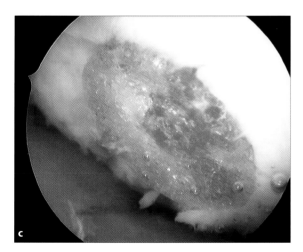

Fig. 43. a Resorbable polymer/calcium implant for osteochondral defects (TruFit©). Note biphasic construction – bone phase (+) and cartilage phase (*). **b** Electron-microscopic picture of a resorbable polymer/calcium implant after contact with spongious blood flow. **c** Arthroscopic view of a resorbable polymer/calcium implant in place after contact with spongious blood flow.

Autologous chondrocyte transplantation (ACT)

Grande and *Peterson* began to transplant autologous chondrocytes in animal experiments in the early 1980's. Their goal was to fill cartilage defects with synthetically active cells to stimulate regeneration of hyaline-like cartilage. Clinical application of ACT to repair full-thickness cartilage defects within the knee joint was first described by *Brittberg et al.* in 1994 (Fig. 44). The technique is as well referred to as autologous chondrocyte implantation (ACI).

▌ **Principle.** Transplantation of autologous chondrocytes into cartilage defects to regenerate hyaline articular cartilage.

▌ **Surgical procedure**
– Perform an arthroscopy to confirm the diagnosis and to measure defect. A cartilage biopsy is taken at the same time. Cartilage samples should be harvested from an area of lesser weight-bearing, i.e. medial or lateral margins of the trochlea (Fig. 45a). In order to achieve standardized cartilage sampling, it is recommended to harvest a 4 mm osteochondral plug from the edge of the intercondylar notch. However, this procedure seems to have higher donor site morbidity.
– Transport of a 200–300 mg cartilage sample to the laboratory occurs under strictly sterile conditions. Different cell culture methods are currently being used. Necessary proteins for cell expansion are gained from serum. Autologous serum offers the advantage of safe immunologic condition in contrast to some serum preparations of animal origin (foetal calf serum). However, the latter offers standardized potency.
Chondrocytes are enzymatically isolated from the matrix under good manufacturing practice and put into monolayer culture. Cells dedifferentiate and proliferate by factor 10–15 until implantation, without being synthetically active.

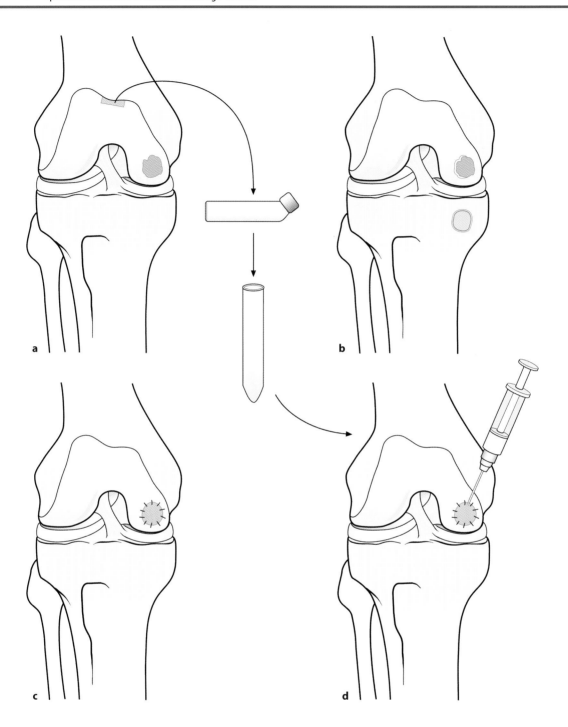

Fig. 44 a–d. Schematic outline of autologous chondrocyte transplantation procedure. **a** Harvesting of a cartilage sample and **b** the periosteal flap. **c** Fixation of periosteal flap with sutures. **d** Injection of chondrocyte suspension.

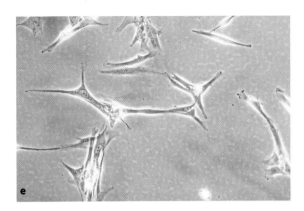

Fig. 44. e Human chondrocytes in monolayer culture for proliferation prior to implantation into a cartilage defect.
f Harvesting of cartilage biopsy from the trochlear rim in arthroscopic view.

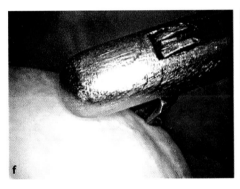
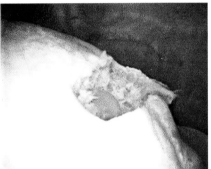

Temporary cryoconservation is feasible. However, potential cell damage is currently being investigated.

– Defects are exposed by a standard arthrotomy. Thorough debridement of degenerative cartilage yet carefully maintaining the integrity of the subchondral bone plate is crucial.

– Defects are debrided until healthy cartilage is reached so a stable defect shoulder can be created. Careful and meticulous hemostasis is critical.

– A periosteal flap of matching size is harvested from the medial tibia which is then sutured onto the defect with the cambium-layer facing down using resorbable thread (5-0/6-0).

– After injection of the chondrocyte-suspension (approx. 0.5 ml) (Fig. 45 b) into the defect, the *bioactive chamber* is sealed with fibrin glue. Cells will adhere to the bottom of the defect within 24–48 h. They redifferentiate and will then synthesize cartilage matrix. 1 million cells per cm^2 of defect area are considered to be sufficient.

■ **Postoperative treatment.** Early functional treatment with immediate mobilisation of the leg using CPM and unlimited range of motion is recommended.

Exception: retropatellar and trochlear defects. For these defects flexion limitation of 60° for two weeks and 90° for the following two weeks has been clinically successful. The knee joint shall be unloaded using sole-contact technique on walking aids for six weeks. For additional support, orthosis' applying valgus or varus stress may be used to unload treated compartments. Sports activities may be started not earlier than 3–4 months after surgery. Aquajogging, swimming or cycling may be performed. Finalization of cartilage regeneration will not be reached until 18–24 months after surgery. This is particularly important in regards to patient expectations, job demands and for preoperative consents. Follow-up examinations shall be performed after 6 months using clinical evaluation and MRI with cartilage-specific sequences (for example 3D FLASH fat suppression according to *Uhl*) (Fig. 47).

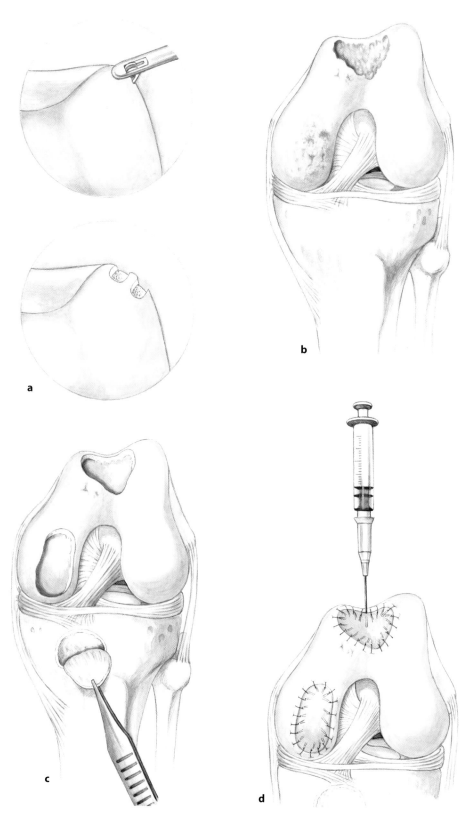

Fig. 45 a–d. Treatment of cartilage lesion using ACT. **a** Harvesting of a cartilage sample, **b** debridement of the defect, **c** harvesting of a periosteal flap (here: from the tibial head), **d** injection of the chondrocyte suspension after suturing the periosteal flap onto the defect site.

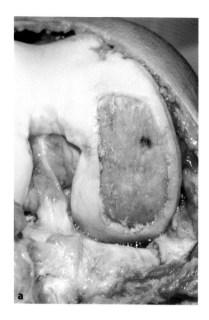

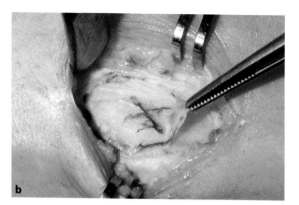

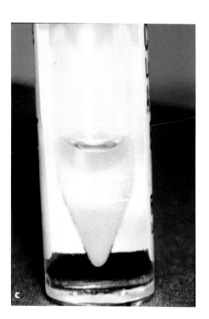

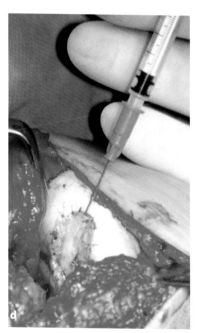

Fig. 46. a Intraoperative view of a large cartilage defect on the femoral condyle after debridement. **b** Harvesting of a periosteal flap from the proximal tibia. The designated intraarticular surface is marked. **c** Autologous chondrocyte suspension (0.7 ml with approx. 10 million cells). **d** Injection of the cell suspension under the periosteal flap into the cartilage defect prior to sealing with fibrin glue. **e** Large cartilage defect on the femoral condyle treated with autologous chondrocyte transplantation.

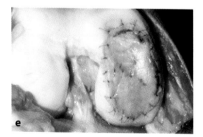

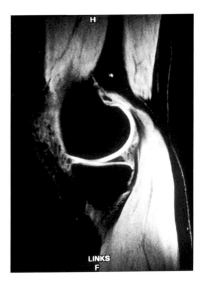

Fig. 47. MRI image of the knee 24 months after ACT on the femoral condyle (sagittal T1 – FLASH fs).

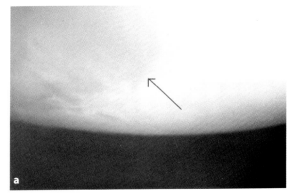

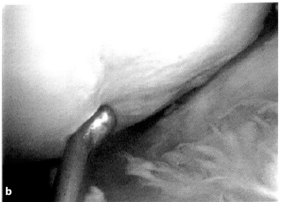

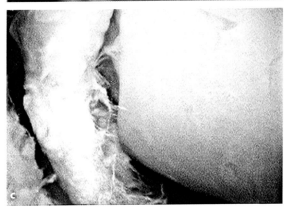

However, detailed qualitative information about the regenerate may currently not be obtained from MRI. Regenerate thickness and potential regenerate hypertrophy may be depicted in reliable manner (Figs. 48, 53).

Second look arthroscopies show quality of lateral regenerate integration (Fig. 54). Indentation measurements depict biomechanical characteristics of the regenerate. Regenerate morphology may only be detected by histological analysis of biopsies (Fig. 55). Biopsies reaching into the subchondral bone using a dedicated biopsy device are recommended (for example Yamshidi, ∅ 1.7 mm).

Autologous chondrocyte transplantation (ACT) – New procedures

Despite satisfying clinical results ACT also shows some technical disadvantages:

▌ Insufficient mechanical stability
▌ Uncertain cell distribution within the defect
▌ Fixation of the periosteal flap with sutures penetrating healthy cartilage
▌ Necessity of intact cartilage shoulder surrounding the defect
▌ Chance of periosteal hypertrophy

Fig. 48 a–c. Arthroscopic view of the femoral condyle after ACT using a periosteal flap. **a** Complete filling of the defect (left top) with smooth surface and good lateral integration within surrounding healthy cartilage (arrow). **b** Complete filling of a cartilage defect showing hypertrophy of the periosteal flap but smooth surface structure. **c** Detachment of a hypertrophic periosteal flap.

Various research groups are therefore in the process of developing three-dimensional cell-carriers to improve techniques for the implantation of articular chondrocytes. Gradual biodegradation of matrices provides space for concomitant formation of neocartilage after a certain time.

The following bioresorbable materials are currently used in various matrices:

▌ Collagens of animal origin (mostly collagen type I and III)
▌ Hyaluronan
▌ Polymers (PLA, PGLA)

These matrices may be fixed by auto-adhesion, with fibrin glue, sutured or anchored transosseously. Biomechanical and preclinical studies showed that the stability of fixation varies tremendously with obvious clinical implications.

Arthroscopic implantation of autologous chondrocytes on bioresorbable cell-carriers is feasible. Using these so-called *scaffolds*, more

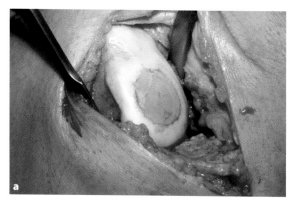

Fig. 49. a Intraoperative view of a cartilage defect on the femoral condyle after implantation of collagen cell carrier (CaRes®) (with kind permission of U. Schneider, München, Germany). **b** Intraoperative view of a cartilage defect on the femoral condyle after autologous chondrocyte transplantation. The periosteal flap is replaced with a collagen I/III membrane (with kind permission of J. Richardson, Oswestry, UK).

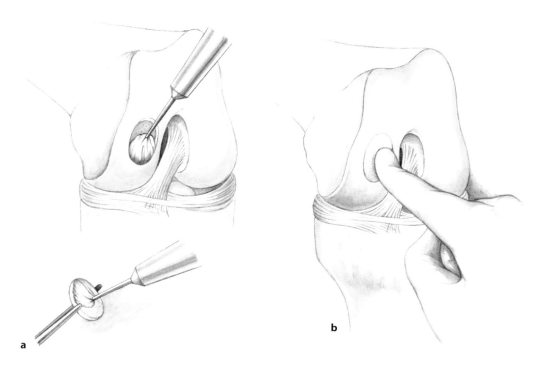

Fig. 50 a, b. Fixation of cell-loaded matrices **a** with fibrin glue and **b** by adhesion only.

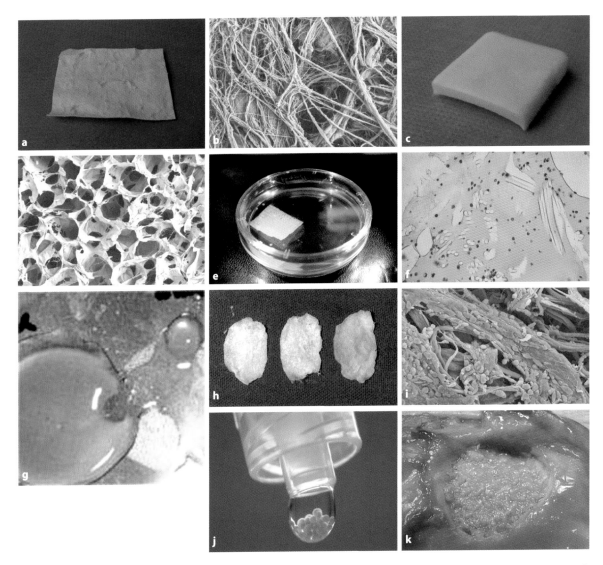

Fig. 51 a–k. Bioresorbable implants serving as cell carriers for autologous chondrocytes: **a** porcine collagen I/III membrane (Chondro-Gide®/Geistlich), **b** ultrastructural image of a porcine collagen I/III membrane, **c** equine collagen fleece (TissueFleece E®/Baxter Bioscience), **d** ultrastructural image of an equine collagen fleece, **e** polyglactid fleece (Bioseed C®/Biotissue Technologies), **f** histological section of a polyglactid fleece with cultured chondrocytes (blue) (with kind permission of M. Sittinger and C. Kaps, Berlin, Germany), **g** murine collagen gel (CaRes®/ArsArthro AG), **h** esterized hyaluronan fleece (Hyalograft®/Fidiapharm), **i** ultrastructural image of a hyaluronan fleece (with kind permission of S. Marlovits, Wien, Austria), **j** condensed chondrocyte pellets (Chondrospheres®/Codon AG), **k** Chondrospheres in a cartilage defect (with kind permission of Codon, Teltow, Germany).

even cell distribution within the defect may be achieved with operative handling being improved at the same time.

Various techniques are currently used for the implantation of matrices (availability may vary from country to country):
▌ After debriding the defect, a size-matching scaffold is sutured or glued into the defect.

Different materials may simply be attached by adhesion forces.
– Hyaluronan Matrix (Fleece) of animal origin/Hyalograft® (Fidia) (Fig. 51 h)
– Collagen-Gel/CaRES® (ArsArthro AG) (Fig. 51 g)
– Collagen matrix/MACT® (CellTec)
– Collagen matrix/MACI® (Genzyme)

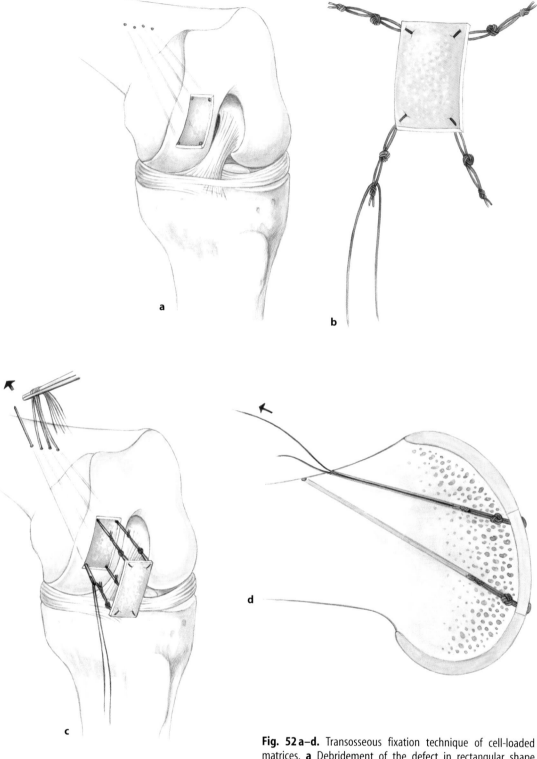

Fig. 52 a–d. Transosseous fixation technique of cell-loaded matrices. **a** Debridement of the defect in rectangular shape and drilling of anchor holes in each corner. **b** Implant pre-armed with resorbable sutures in every corner (woven, 2-0) using special knotting techniques. **c** Insertion of pre-armed implant into the defect. **d** Principle of transosseous anchoring of the implant by press fit-insertion of knots into holes.

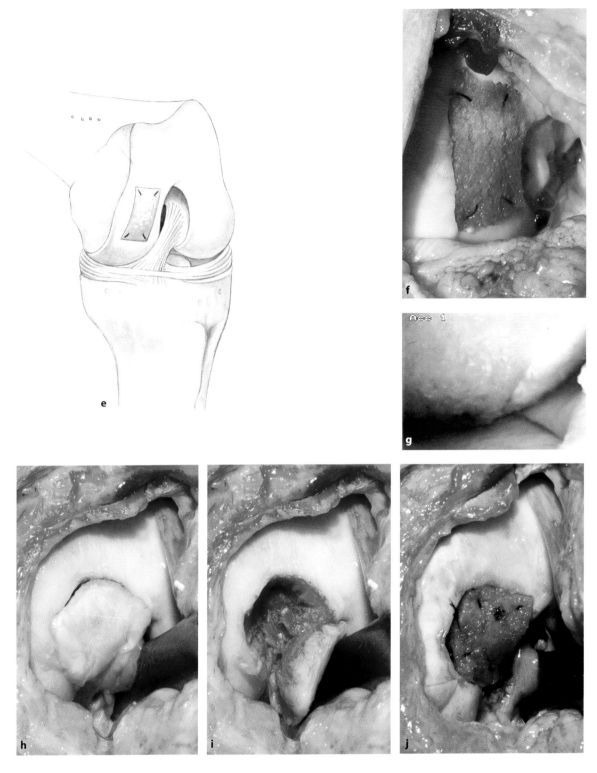

Fig. 52. e Transosseously fixed implant in-situ. **f** Intraoperative view of a cartilage defect on the femoral condyle after implantation of a cell-loaded polymer fleece (Bioseed C®). **g** Arthroscopic view of a femoral condyle after arthroscopic implantation of a cell-loaded polymer fleece. Large osteochondral defect of the femoral condyle (**h**), after grafting with autologous spongious bone (**i**) and matrix augmented ACT (**j**).

∎ After exact determination of the defect size a matching implant is prepared. The implant will then be pre-armed with resorbable threads (Vicryl) which are to be knotted using a special technique. Anchoring holes will be placed anterogradely or tibially using a guide instrument. After insertion of pulling threads the pre-armed matrix is anchored within the defect by pulling the knots into the holes (Fig. 51 a–g).

– Polyglactin/poly-p-dioxanon Fleece/Bioseed-C® (Biotissue-Technologies)

∎ Stable matrices enable a fast and stable but more costly fixation with intraosseous pins (Smart Nail©).

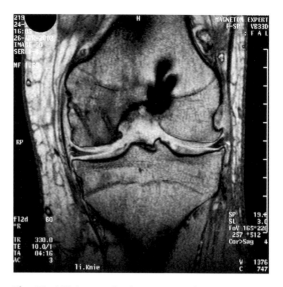

Fig. 53. MRI image of a knee 12 months after implantation of a polymer fleece with autologous chondrocytes. Canals from transosseous anchoring are barely to identify.

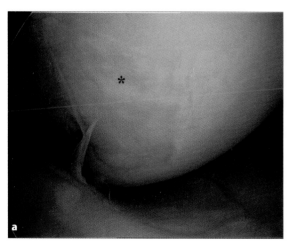

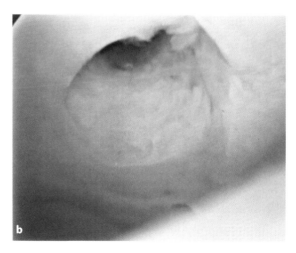

Fig. 54 a, b. a Arthroscopic view of a femoral condyle 9 months after implantation of a polymer fleece with autologous chondrocytes (*). **b** Transplantation site after autologous chondrocyte transplantation and core biopsy with a Yamshidi needle.

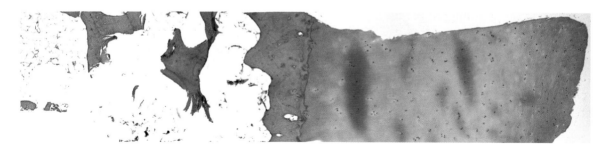

Fig. 55. Histological section of a osteochondral biopsy 9 months after implantation of a polymer fleece with autologous chondrocytes (in collaboration with J. Schwarzkopf, Freiburg, Germany).

Correctional osteotomies

Juxtaarticular correctional osteotomies for the treatment of axial malalignments are to be considered as indirect treatment options in cartilage therapy. Varus and valgus deformities of the knee are the most common amongst axial malalignments. For further information about deformities of ankle, elbow and hip joint refer to specific literature covering these entities.

Treatment of cartilaginous lesions may only be successful with a given physiologic axial alignment of the joint. Thus, malalignments ought to be corrected prior to or at the same time a dedicated cartilage repair procedure.

Various techniques have been established and used successfully. High tibial valgisation osteotomy is the most commonly performed procedure since varus deformities of the knee is most common. One has to distinguish between *closed wedge* and *open wedge* techniques, which shall be outlined briefly in the following paragraph. Different sets of instruments for osteosynthesis are currently available.

∎ **Principle.** Unloading of lesioned or regenerating articular cartilage by means of juxtaarticular correctional osteotomy to restore physiologic mechanical axis.

∎ **Indications.** Varus and valgus deformities of the knee joint with medialization or lateralization of the physiologic mechanical axis.

∎ **Diagnostics.** For both diagnosis finding and procedure planning long leg standing films including hip and ankle joint are essential. Short films are sufficient for the lateral view. The extent of malalignment may then be measured using drawings based on the standing AP views or by digital analysis. Necessary corrections may be determined according to those measurements.

In case of concomitant osteoarthritic changes in the contralateral compartment or in the femoropatellar joint one should refrain from performing an osteotomy. Total knee arthroplasty shall be taken into consideration instead.

Surgical procedure

Closed-wedge technique

Performance of a fibular osteotomy. A closed wedge high tibial valgisation osteotomy is, in most cases, not feasible without a fibula osteotomy, since the fibula inhibits lateral approach and valgisation. One has to pay special attention to the potential risk of damaging the peroneal nerve. It is located dorsally of the fibular head.

Different techniques may be used:
∎ Extraction of a bone cylinder (1 cm) from the medial third of the fibula using an additional 5 cm skin incision.
∎ Fibular head osteotomy: this technique avoids an additional skin incision but bears the risk of causing nerve palsy.
∎ Tibiofibular disruption: the tibiofibular joint is disrupted using a chisel which will allow mobilization of the fibula. In case of a correction angle $> 10°$ this technique will not provide sufficient fibular mobility.
∎ Exposure of the ventrolateral tibial head using a curvilinear or straight incision.
∎ Determination of osteotomy level (usually under fluoroscopy).
∎ Extraction of a bone wedge with lateral basis. Width of the basis depends on preoperative planning. Two different techniques are currently being used:
  – Wedge-shaped osteotomy using an oscillating saw which is available with angle measuring devices (Fig. 56 a).
    Cave: Complete transsection of the medial cortical bone and the periosteum may result in instability of the medial column during postoperative rehabilitation.
  – A wedge is created by using drill bits of increasing size until pre-determined width of the wedge basis is reached. Medial cortical bone is then perforated using a 2 mm drill bit. This procedure offers the advantage of increased rotational stability due to

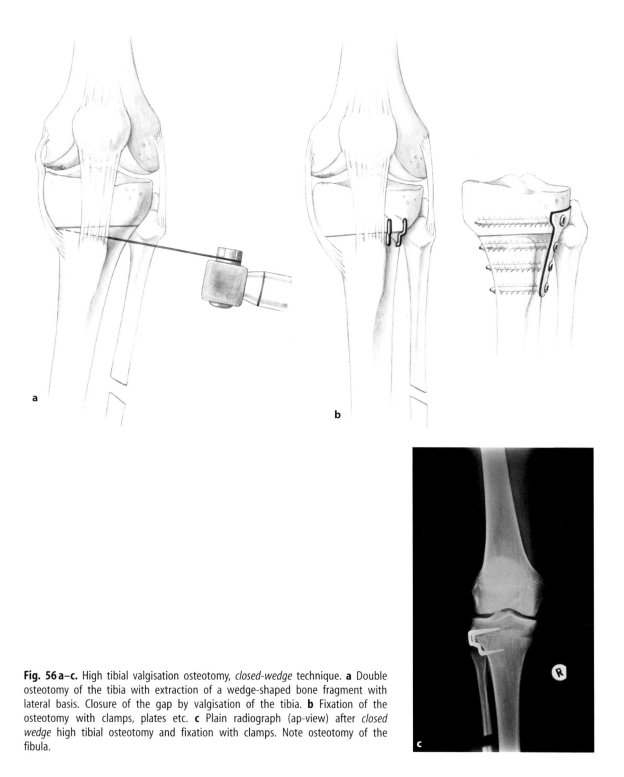

Fig. 56 a–c. High tibial valgisation osteotomy, *closed-wedge* technique. **a** Double osteotomy of the tibia with extraction of a wedge-shaped bone fragment with lateral basis. Closure of the gap by valgisation of the tibia. **b** Fixation of the osteotomy with clamps, plates etc. **c** Plain radiograph (ap-view) after *closed wedge* high tibial osteotomy and fixation with clamps. Note osteotomy of the fibula.

rough surfaces of osteotomy levels. Lateral defect is then closed by valgisation of the tibia. Stable osteosynthesis is achieved using Giebel-plates, T-plates or Blount's staples (Fig. 56 b, c).

– A ventrally shifted wedge basis may allow increased extension in some exceptional cases, which might help to ease femoropatellar pain post-surgery. One has to take into consideration that varisation of the mechanical axis affects patella tracking, i.e. patella tracking will be lateralized. Patients usually benefit from this but may also sense pain thereafter.

Open-wedge technique

Open wedge technique uses a medially opening osteotomy.
▌ Exposure of the ventromedial tibial head.
▌ Oblique, laterally inclining, subtotal osteotomy using an oscillating saw under fluoroscopic control (Fig. 57).
▌ Opening of the osteotomy through valgisation of the tibia to the predetermined extent.

▌ Filling of the wedge-shaped osteotomy defect using autologous spongiosa or bone substitute.

Special plates with wedge-shaped spacers of increasing size are available to keep osteotomy basis open until bony reconstitution is reached. In case of instability of the medial collateral ligament due to an osteotomy proximal of the tibial insertion of the MCL, insertion of a cortico-spongioseal wedge from the iliac crest usually provides sufficient stability. Additional osteosynthesis is not necessary in most cases (Fig. 57b). Bioresorbable implants (spacers) and new plates offering angular stability are also available.

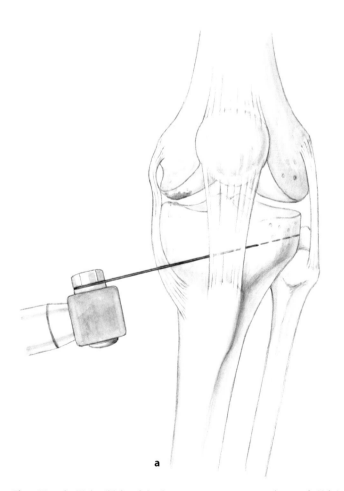

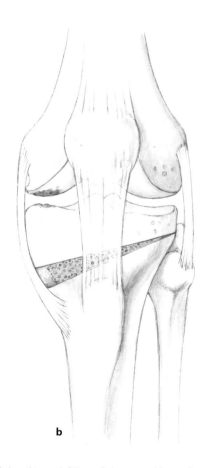

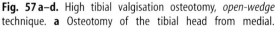

Fig. 57 a–d. High tibial valgisation osteotomy, *open-wedge* technique. **a** Osteotomy of the tibial head from medial. **b** Valgisation of the tibia and filling of the gap with autologous bone or bone substitute.

▮ **Combination procedures.** If juxtaarticular osteotomies are necessary in addition to other surgical procedures of the same knee joint it is often useful to perform those at the same time in order to offer the shortest possible rehabilitation to the patient. Cartilage repair procedures – arthroscopic or arthrotomic – shall be performed prior to the osteotomy to avoid intraoperatively applied mechanical stress of hyperflexion upon a fresh osteotomy site.

In case an osteotomy is performed in combination with an ACL-reconstruction one should first drill holes for the graft and then insert the graft itself *after* completion of the osteotomy. Slight revision of the tibial hole might be necessary.

Rare cases, especially valgus deformities, require performance of a distal femoral (supracondylar) osteotomy using angled blade plates. Details of this considerably more lavish and more difficult surgical procedure shall be drawn from dedicated text books.

Future perspectives include use of navigation systems for more precise preoperative planning.

▮ **Postoperative treatment.** High tibial osteotomies should be primarily stable enough for passive motion and early range of motion exercise. Active, load-bearing extension should be avoided due to pull of the patellar tendon distally of the osteotomy level.

Unloading of the operated limb with toe touch weight bearing only is recommended for at least six weeks. Fixed-angle stabilisation with modern implants allow early weight bearing after 2 weeks. Depending on radiographic controls longer unloading periods of up to three months may be necessary.

▮ **Pitfalls**

▮ Intraoperative fracture (Fig. 57 d).

▮ Fixation (osteosynthesis) failure
Temporary cast-immobilization should be used before considering revision surgery.

▮ Compartment syndrome
Postoperative, non-segmental loss of sensibility and palsies of the foot may be symptoms of a compartment syndrome. Pressure measurements within the different compartments can provide additional information to secure diagnosis. This is an easy-to-perform and cost-effective procedure. In doubtful cases large scale fasciotomy is the only way to prevent irreversible muscle and nerve damage.

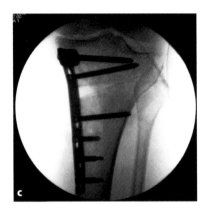

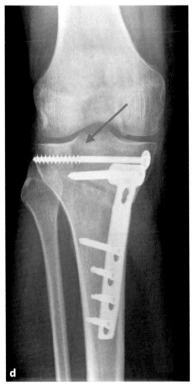

Fig. 57 c, d. Plain radiograph (ap-view) after *open wedge* high tibial osteotomy and fixation with Tomofix® plate (**c**). The osteotomy gap is NOT filled. Note fracture or the tibial joint surface after correction (arrow) (**d**).

▌ Lesion of the peroneal nerve
Immediate postoperative weakness or palsy of the extensor hallucis muscle is commonly caused by affection of the peroneal nerve. Malfunction of this particular muscle does not necessarily imply sharp nerve damage. Intraoperative development of heat, mechanical alteration by surgical instruments or haematoma formation may be causes of the described muscle malfunction. Special neurological examination may contribute to clarify the diagnosis and also allow prognosis.

▌ Malunion
In case of delayed union or nonunion of the osteotomy area beyond a period of three months, extracorporeal shock wave therapy has shown promising results. Failure of this conservative approach should be followed by revision surgery including debridement of the osteotomy surfaces and bone grafting using autologous spongiosa.

▌ Failure of fixation or fixation device
Accidental overload may result in fixation failure with the imperative need of revision surgery.

▌ Slow re-varisation or -valgisation
Rare cases show gradual loss of axial correction due to osteoporotic changes. These cases also require revision surgery to prevent further structural damage. Temporary use of orthosis applying valgus or varus stress may be helpful.

▌ **Advantages**
– Joint saving procedure
– High clinical acceptance
– Low costs (depending on the implant).

▌ **Disadvantages**
– Demanding surgical procedure
– Considerable risks
– Long rehabilitation (depending on the implant).

Implantation of non-resorbable cartilage replacements

Various synthetic materials have been used in the past to restore cartilage surfaces and decrease friction and to repair focal cartilage injuries. Silicon injections were for example performed in the 1960s. Various techniques are nowadays introduced promising dramatic success and efficacy.

Carbon fibre

Carbon fibre pads were used for the reconstruction of joint surfaces in England in the early 1980s. Carbon fibre plugs are nowadays available for the treatment of articular cartilage defects.

▌ **Principle.** Carbon fibre constructs shall serve as scaffolds to promote formation of fibrous regenerates.

▌ **Surgical procedure.** Implantation is usually performed arthroscopically. Defects are to be debrided prior to implantation. Holes are then drilled within the defect area matching the dimensions of the carbon fibre plugs (12.5×3 mm). Special application devices help to insert plugs into holes. Upper ends of the plugs shall be congruent with the bone surface (Fig. 59). Carbon fibre plugs swell immediately after implantation fixing them securely within the hole. Penetration of subchondral bone in this manner shall promote migration of cells into the defect to form fibrocartilage (Fig. 58). In comparison with microfracture techniques carbon fibre plugs supposedly provide prolonged exposure of subchondral bone for extended diffusion of bioactive substances into the lesion. Distance between plugs should be 5–7 mm.

▌ **Pitfalls.** Plugs must not reach above the level of subchondral bone to avoid damage of the corresponding joint surface risking release of carbon fibre debris.

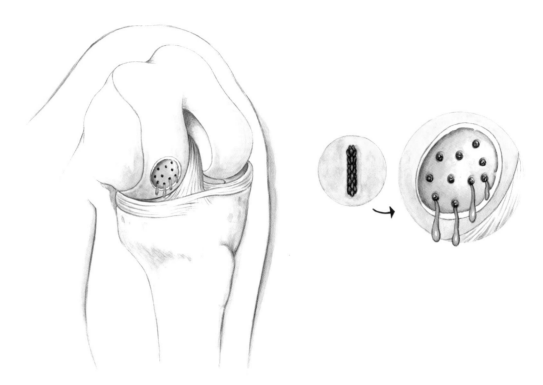

Fig. 58. Treatment of a femoral cartilage defect with carbon plugs (Arthrocarb®).

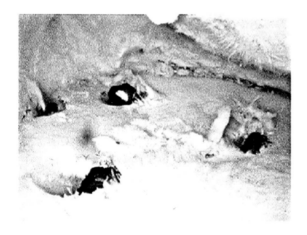

Fig. 59. Arthroscopic view of a large osteoarthritic lesion on the tibial plateau after implantation of carbon plugs.

▌ **Postoperative treatment.** Physiotherapy with unlimited range of motion immediately after surgery. Unloading of the operated limb for at least six weeks with optional use of an orthosis for compartmental unloading.

▌ **Advantages**
– Arthroscopic technique.

▌ **Disadvantages**
– Non-biologic approach using non-resorbable material (Fig. 60b)
– Risk of inflammatory synovial response
– Considerably high costs (approx. 80 €/plug)
– Risk of secondary complications when implanting total knee endoprosthesis. Extremely stable carbon fibre plugs grossly interfere with the preparation of the bone with the oscillating saw (Fig. 60a).

▌ **Hemi cap.** A Cr-Co-Mo/titanium contoured articular prosthetic device (HemiCAP®) was designed to restore osteo-cartilaginous defects in various joints. An articular resurfacing component and a cancellous taper post mate together via a taper interlock to provide stable and immobile fixation of the implant and stress bearing contact at the bone/prosthetic interface. Various implants are available to ensure congruity of the cartilage surface.

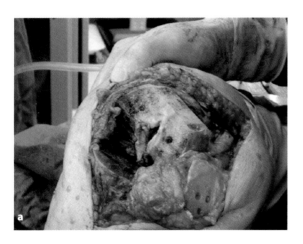

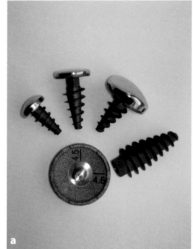

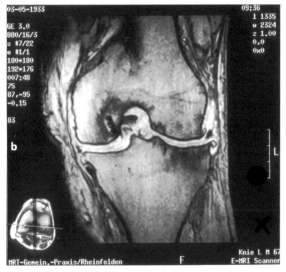

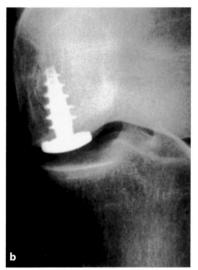

Fig. 60. a Intraoperative view of a knee joint after implantation of carbon plugs, prior to total knee arthroplasty (with kind permission of H.R. Henche, Rheinfelden, Germany). **b** MRI image of a knee joint after implantation of carbon plugs showing a zone osteolysis in subchondral bone around the plug.

Fig. 61. a Modular implants for treatment of full thickness cartilage defects (hemicap®/Arthrosurface). **b** Plain radiograph showing metallic implant (hemicap®) anchored in the femoral condyle.

Additional Reading

Anderson AF, Pagnani MJ (1997) Osteochondritis Dissecans of the Femoral Condyles. Am J Sports Med 25:830–834.

Baker B, Becker RO, Spadaro J (2001) A study of electrochemical enhancement of articular cartilage repair. Clin Orthop 102:251–267.

Bentley G, Greer RBI (1971) Homotransplantation of isolated epiphyseal and articular cartilage chondrocytes into joint surfaces of rabbits. Nature 230:385–388.

Bentley G, Biant LC, Carrington RW, Akmal M, Goldberg A, Williams AM, Skinner JA, Pringle J (2003) A prospective, randomised comparison of autologous chondrocyte implantation versus mosaicplasty for osteochondral defects in the knee. J Bone Joint Surg Br 85:223–230.

Bobic V (1996) Arthroscopic osteochondral autograft transplantation in anterior cruciate ligament reconstruction: a preliminary clinical study. Knee Surg Sports Traumatol Arthrosc 3:262–264.

Brittberg M, Lindahl A, Nilsson A, Ohlsson C, Isaksson O, Peterson L (1994) Treatment of deep cartilage defects in the knee with autologous chondrocyte transplantation. N Engl J Med 331:889–895.

Brittberg M, Faxen E, Peterson L (1994) Carbon fiber scaffolds in the treatment of early knee osteoarthritis. A prospective 4-year followup of 37 patients. Clin Orthop 155–164.

Brittberg M, Winalski CS (2003) Evaluation of cartilage injuries and repair. J Bone Joint Surg Am 85-A (Suppl 2):58–69.

Buckwalter JA, Mankin HJ (1997) Articular cartilage – Part I. J Bone Joint Surg 79-A:600–611.

Clegg DO, Reda DJ, Harris CL, Klein MA, O'Dell JR, Hooper MM, Bradley JD, Bingham CO 3rd, Weisman MH, Jackson CG, Lane NE, Cush JJ, Moreland LW, Schumacher HR Jr, Oddis CV, Wolfe F, Molitor JA, Yocum DE, Schnitzer TJ, Furst DE, Sawitzke AD, Shi H, Brandt KD, Moskowitz RW, Williams HJ (2006) Glucosamine, chondroitin sulfate, and the two in combination for painful knee osteoarthritis. N Engl J Med 354(8):795–808.

Dorotka R, Windberger U, Macfelda K, Bindreiter U, Toma C, Nehrer S (2005) Repair of articular cartilage defects treated by microfracture and a three-dimensional collagen matrix. Biomaterials 26(17):3617–3629.

Driesang IM, Hunziker EB (2000) Delamination rates of tissue flaps used in articular cartilage repair. J Orthop Res 18:909–911.

Drobnic M, Radosavljevic D, Ravnik D, Pavlovcic V, Hribernik M (2006) Comparison of four techniques for the fixation of a collagen scaffold in the human cadaveric knee. Osteoarthritis Cartilage 14(4):337–344.

Erggelet C, Steinwachs MR, Reichelt A (2000) The operative treatment of full thickness cartilage defects in the knee joint with autologous chondrocyte transplantation. Saudi Med J 21:715–721.

Erggelet C, Sittinger M, Lahm A (2003) The arthroscopic implantation of autologous chondrocytes for the treatment of full-thickness cartilage defects of the knee joint. Arthroscopy 19:108–110.

Erggelet C, Neumann K, Endres M, Haberstroh K, Sittinger M, Kaps C (2007) Regeneration of ovine articular cartilage defects by cell-free polymer-based implants. Biomaterials 28(36):5570–5580.

Frisbie DD, Oxford JT, Southwood L, Trotter GW, Rodkey WG, Steadman JR, Goodnight JL, McIlwraith CW (2003) Early events in cartilage repair after subchondral bone microfracture. Clin Orthop 215–227.

Grande DA, Pitman MI, Peterson L, Menche D, Klein M (1989) The repair of experimentally produced defects in rabbit articular cartilage by autologous chondrocyte transplantation. J Orthop Res 7:208–218.

Hangody L, Kish G, Karpati Z, Udvarhelyi I, Szigeti I, Bely M (1998) Mosaicplasty for the treatment of articular cartilage defects: application in clinical practice. Orthopedics 21:751–756.

Hangody L, Fules P (2003) Autologous osteochondral mosaicplasty for the treatment of full-thickness defects of weight-bearing joints: ten years of experimental and clinical experience. J Bone Joint Surg Am 85-A (Suppl 2):25–32.

Henderson I, Lavigne P, Valenzuela H, Oakes B (2007) Autologous chondrocyte implantation: superior biologic properties of hyaline cartilage repairs. Clin Orthop Relat Res 455:253–261.

Homandberg GA, Guo D, Ray LM, Ding L (2006) Mixtures of glucosamine and chondroitin sulfate reverse fibronectin fragment mediated damage to cartilage more effectively than either agent alone. Osteoarthritis Cartilage 14(8):793–806.

Horas U, Pelinkovic D, Herr G, Aigner T, Schnettler R (2003) Autologous chondrocyte implantation and osteochondral cylinder transplantation in cartilage repair of the knee joint. A prospective, comparative trial. J Bone Joint Surg Am 85-A: 185–192.

Hubbard MJS (1996) Articular debridement vs. washout for degeneration of the medial femoral condyle. J Bone Joint Surg 78-B:217–219.

Hunziker EB (1999) Biologic repair of articular cartilage. Defect models in experimental animals and matrix requirements. Clin Orthop 135–146.

Imhoff AB, Burkart A, Ottl GM (1999) Transfer of the posterior femoral condyle. First experience with a salvage operation. Orthopäde 28:45–51.

Jerosch J, Filler T, Peuker E (2001) Theoretische und experimentelle Grundlagen sowie Operationstechnik der T-F-Plastik. In: Erggelet C, Steinwachs MR (eds) Gelenkknorpeldefekte. Steinkopff, Darmstadt, 109–123.

Johnson LL (1986) Arthroscopic abrasion arthroplasty historical and pathologic perspective: present status. Arthroscopy 2:54–69.

Johnson LL, Uitvlugt G, Austin MD, Detrisac DA, Johnson C (1990) Osteochondritis dissecans of the knee: arthroscopic compression screw fixation. Arthroscopy 6:179–189.

Knecht S, Erggelet C, Endres M, Sittinger M, Kaps C, Stussi E (2007) Mechanical testing of fixation techniques for scaffold-based tissue-engineered grafts. J Biomed Mater Res B Appl Biomater.

Knutsen G, Drogset JO, Engebretsen L, Grontvedt T, Isaksen V, Ludvigsen TC et al (2007) A randomized trial comparing autologous chondrocyte implantation with microfracture. Findings at five years. J Bone Joint Surg Am 89(10):2105–2112.

Kreuz PC, Steinwachs MR, Erggelet C, Krause SJ, Konrad G, Uhl M, Sudkamp N (2006) Results after microfracture of full-thickness chondral defects in different compartments in the knee. Osteoarthritis Cartilage 14(11):1119–1125.

Levy AS, Lohnes J, Sculley S, LeCroy M, Garret W (1996) Chondral delamination of knee in soccer players. Am J Sports Med 24:634–639.

Lubowitz JH, Verdonk PC, Reid JB 3rd, Verdonk R (2007) Meniscus allograft transplantation: a current concepts review. Knee Surg Sports Traumatol Arthrosc 15(5):476–492.

Lysholm J, Gillquist J (1982) Evaluation of knee ligament surgery results with special emphasis on use of a scoring scale. Am J Sports Med 10:150–154.

Lyyra T, Kiviranta I, Vaatainen U, Helminen HJ, Jurvelin JS (1999) In vivo characterization of indentation stiffness of articular cartilage in the normal human knee. J Biomed Mater Res 48:482–487.

Mainil-Varlet P, Aigner T, Brittberg M, Bullough P, Hollander A, Hunziker E, Kandel R, Nehrer S, Pritzker K, Roberts S, Stauffer E, International Cartilage Repair Society (2003) Histological assessment of cartilage repair: a report by the Histology

Endpoint Committee of the International Cartilage Repair Society (ICRS). J Bone Joint Surg Am 85-A (Suppl 2):45–57.

Mandelbaum BR, Browne JE, Fu F, Micheli L, Mosely JB Jr, Erggelet C, Minas T, Peterson L (1998) Articular cartilage lesions of the knee. Am J Sports Med 26:853–861.

Mandelbaum B, Browne JE, Fu F, Micheli LJ, Moseley JB Jr, Erggelet C, Anderson AF (2007) Treatment outcomes of autologous chondrocyte implantation for full-thickness articular cartilage defects of the trochlea. Am J Sports Med 35(6):915–921.

Mankin HJ, Dorfman H, Lippiello L, Zarins A (1971) Biochemical and metabolic abnormalities in articular cartilage from osteo-arthritic human hips. II. Correlation of morphology with biochemical and metabolic data. J Bone Joint Surg Am 53:523–537.

Messner K, Gillquist J (1996) Cartilage repair. A critical review. Acta Orthop Scand 67:523–529.

Micheli LJ, Browne JE, Erggelet C, Fu F, Mandelbaum B, Moseley JB, Zurakowski D (2001) Autologous chondrocyte implantation of the knee: multicenter experience and minimum 3-year follow-up. Clin J Sport Med 11:223–228.

Micheli LJ, Moseley JB, Anderson AF, Browne JE, Erggelet C, Arciero R, Fu FH, Mandelbaum BR (2006) Articular cartilage defects of the distal femur in children and adolescents: treatment with autologous chondrocyte implantation. J Pediatr Orthop 26(4):455–460.

Mithoefer K, Scopp JM, Mandelbaum BR (2007) Articular Cartilage Repair in Athletes. Instr Course Lect 56:457–468.

Moseley JB, O'Malley K, Petersen NJ, Menke TJ, Brody BA, Kuykendall DH, Hollingsworth JC, Ashton CM, Wray NP (2002) A controlled trial of arthroscopic surgery for osteoarthritis of the knee. N Engl J Med 347(2):81–88.

Nehrer S, Breinan HA, Ramappa A, Shortkroff S, Young G, Minas T, Sledge CB, Yannas IV, Spector M (1997) Canine chondrocytes seeded in type I and type II collagen implants investigated in vitro. J Biomed Mater Res 38:95–104.

Nehrer S, Breinan HA, Ramappa A, Hsu HP, Minas T, Shortkroff S, Sledge CB, Yannas IV, Spector M (1998) Chondrocyte-seeded collagen matrices implanted in a chondral defect in a canine model. Biomaterials 19:2313–2328.

O'Driscoll SW, Keeley FW, Salter RB (1986) The chondrogenic potential of free autogenous periosteal grafts for biological resurfacing of major full-thickness defects in joint surfaces under the influence of continuous passive motion. An experimental investigation in the rabbit. J Bone Joint Surg Am 68:1017–1035.

Ossendorf C, Kaps C, Kreuz PC, Burmester GR, Sittinger M, Erggelet C (2007) Treatment of posttraumatic and focal osteoarthritic cartilage defects of the knee with autologous polymer-based three-dimensional chondrocyte grafts: 2-year clinical results. Arthritis Res Ther 9(2):R41 [Epub ahead of print].

Outerbridge HK, Outerbridge AR, Outerbridge RE (1995) The use of a lateral patellar autologous graft for the repair of a large osteochondral defect in the knee. J Bone Joint Surg Am 77:65–72.

Perka C, Sittinger M, Schultz O, Spitzer RS, Schlenzka D, Burmester GR (2000) Tissue engineered cartilage repair using cryopreserved and noncryopreserved chondrocytes. Clin Orthop 245–254.

Peterson L, Minas T, Brittberg M, Nilsson A, Sjogren-Jansson E, Lindahl A (2000) Two- to 9-year outcome after autologous chondrocyte transplantation of the knee. Clin Orthop 212–234.

Peterson L, Minas T, Brittberg M, Lindahl A (2003) Treatment of osteochondritis dissecans of the knee with autologous chondrocyte transplantation: results at two to ten years. J Bone Joint Surg Am 85-A (Suppl 2):17–24.

Potter HG, Foo LF (2006) Magnetic resonance imaging of articular cartilage: trauma, degeneration repair. Am J Sports Med 34(4):661–677.

Pridie KH (1959) A method of resurfacing arthritic knee joints. J Bone Joint Surg 41-B:618–619.

Radin EL, Ehrlich MG, Chernack R, Abernethy P, Paul IL, Rose RM (1978) Effect of repetitive impulsive loading on the knee joints of rabbits. Clin Orthop 288–293.

Reddy S, Pedowitz DI, Parekh SG, Sennett BJ, Okereke E (2007) The morbidity associated with osteochondral harvest from asymptomatic knees for the treatment of osteochondral lesions of the talus. Am J Sports Med 35(1):80–85.

Rodkey WG, Steadman JR, Li ST (1999) A clinical study of collagen meniscus implants to restore the injured meniscus. Clin Orthop 281–292.

Saris DB, Vanlauwe J, Victor J, Haspl M, Bohnsack M, Fortems Y, et al (2008) Characterized chondrocyte implantation results in better structural repair when treating symptomatic cartilage defects of the knee in a randomized controlled trial versus microfracture. Am J Sports Med 36(2):235–246.

Sittinger M, Reitzel D, Dauner M, Hierlemann H, Hammer C, Kastenbauer E, Planck H, Burmester GR, Bujia J (1996) Resorbable polyesters in cartilage engineering: affinity and biocompatibility of polymer fiber structures to chondrocytes. J Biomed Mater Res 33:57–63.

Smith GD, Taylor J, Almqvist KF, Erggelet C, Knutsen G, Garcia Portabella M, Smith T, Richardson JB (2005) Arthroscopic assessment of cartilage repair: a validation study of 2 scoring systems. Arthroscopy 21(12):1462–1467.

Steadman JR, Rodkey WG, Briggs KK, Rodrigo JJ (1999) The microfracture technic in the management of complete cartilage defects in the knee joint. Orthopäde 28:26–32.

Steadman JR, Ramappa AJ, Maxwell RB, Briggs KK (2007) An arthroscopic treatment regimen for osteoarthritis of the knee. Arthroscopy 23(9):948–955.

Trattnig S, Millington SA, Szomolanyi P, Marlovits S (2007) MR imaging of osteochondral grafts and autologous chondrocyte implantation. Eur Radiol 17(1):103–118.

Uhl M, Allmann KH, Tauer U, Laubenberger J, Adler CP, Ihling C, Langer M (1998) Comparison of MR sequences in quantifying in vitro cartilage degeneration in osteoarthritis of the knee. Br J Radiol 71:291–296.

Uhl M (2001) Magnetresonanztomographie des hyalinen Gelenkknorpels. In: Erggelet C, Steinwachs MR (eds) Gelenkknorpeldefekte. Steinkopff, Darmstadt, 71–81.

Wagner H (1974) Operative Behandlung der Osteochondritis dissecans des Kniegelenkes. Z Orthop 98:333–355.

Appendix

Scores for the evaluation of therapy results after treatment of articular cartilage defects (selection)

▌ ICRS
ICRS evaluation.pdf

▌ KOOS
KOOSGuide2003.pdf
KOOSScoringfile.xls

▌ Modified Cincinnati Score (Cartilage Repair Registry)

▌ Lysholm
lysholm.doc

▌ Tegner

▌ Freiburg Ankle Score (FAS)
ankle score.doc

ICRS Cartilage Injury Evaluation Package

Consists of two parts:

A: PATIENT PART:
ICRS Injury questionnaire
The IKDC Subjective Knee Evaluation Form-2000

B: SURGEONS PART
ICRS Knee Surgery History Registration
IKDC KneeExamination form-2000
ICRS- Articular cartilage injury mapping system
ICRS-Articular cartilage injury classification
ICRS-Osteochondritis dissecans classification
ICRS-Cartilage Repair Assessment system

The ICRS Clinical Cartilage Injury Evaluation system-2000 was developed during ICRS 2000 Standards Workshop at Schloss Münchenwiler, Switzerland, January 27-30, 2000 and further discussed during the 3rd ICRS Meeting in Göteborg, Sweden, Friday April 28, 2000.
The participants in the Clinical Münchenwiler Evaluation Group were as follows:

Chairman Mats Brittberg, Sweden
Paolo Aglietti, Italy
Ralph Gambardella, USA
Laszlo Hangody, Hungary
Hans Jörg Hauselmann, Switzerland
Roland P Jakob, Switzerland
David Levine, USA
Stefan Lohmander, Sweden
Bert R Mandelbaum, USA
Lars Peterson, Sweden
Hans-Ulrich Staubli, Switzerland

There was a discussion regarding the use of IKDC-1999 vs KOOS (**K**nee Injury and **O**steoarthritis **O**utcome **S**core). The decision in Göteborg was to continue with IKDC (IKDC representatives: A. Anderson, R. Jakob, H.-U. Stäubli) but there will also be comparative studies with the KOOS (http://www.koos.nu/)

The clinical evaluation system can also be combined with the ICRS Imaging Protocol as well as the ICRS Biomechanical Protocol

Comments on the ICRS Cartilage Evaluation forms to: mats.brittberg@telia.com

(with kind permission from International Cartilage Repair Society)

ICRS – CARTILAGE INJURY STANDARD EVALUATION FORM-2000
PATIENTS PART

Patient Name:_____

Birthdate : Day_____ **Month**_____**Year**_____

Street:_____ _____ Zip:_____Town:_____Country:_____

Phone:_____E -mail:_____

Gender:_____

Height:_____cm Weight:_____Kg

Examiner:_____Date of examination:_____

Localisation:

Involved knee: Right ____ Left____

Opposite knee: Normal__ Nearly Normal__Abnormal__Severely abnormal__

Onset of symptoms

(date):_____ Gradual:_____Acute:_____

Etiology/Cause of injury:

Activity at injury:

Activity of daily living:_____Sports_____

Traffic_____Type of vehicle_____ Work_____

Activity-level:	before Injury	Just now prior to surgery
I: high competitive sportsman/woman	yes___No___	yes___No___
II: well-trained and frequently sporting:	yes___No___	yes___No___
III: sporting sometimes	yes___No___	yes___No___
IV: Non-sporting	yes___No___	yes___No___

Functional status

I: I can do everything that I want to do with my joint
II: I can do nearly everything that I want to do with my joint
III: I am restricted and a lot of things that I want to do with my joint are not possible
IV: I am very restricted and I can do almost nothing with my joint without severe pain and disability

Preinjury:	I___II___III___IV___
Just prior to surgery	I___II___III___IV___
Present activity level ˙	I___II___III___IV___

IKDC CURRENT HEALTH ASSESSMENT FORM *
Patients Part:

Your Full Name _____

Your Date of Birth _____/_____/_____
                         Day   Month   Year

Today's Date _____/_____/_____
                    Day   Month   Year

1. In general, would you say your health is:

   ❑ Excellent
   ❑ Very good
   ❑ Good
   ❑ Fair
   ❑ Poor

2. Compared to one year ago, how would you rate your health in general now?

   ❑ Much better now than 1 year ago
   ❑ Somewhat better now than 1 year ago
   ❑ About the same as 1 year ago
   ❑ Somewhat worse now than 1 year ago
   ❑ Much worse now than 1 year ago

3. The following items are about activities you might do during a typical day. Does your health now limit you in these activities? If so, how much?

		Yes, Limited A Lot	Yes, Limited A Little	No, Not Limited At All
a.	Vigorous activities, such as running, lifting heavy objects, participating in strenuous sports	❑	❑	❑
b.	Moderate activities, such as moving a table, pushing a vacuum cleaner, bowling, or playing golf	❑	❑	❑
c.	Lifting or carrying groceries	❑	❑	❑
d.	Climbing several flights of stairs	❑	❑	❑
e.	Climbing one flight of stairs	❑	❑	❑
f.	Bending, kneeling or stooping	❑	❑	❑
g.	Walking more than a mile	❑	❑	❑
h.	Walking several blocks	❑	❑	❑
i.	Walking one block	❑	❑	❑
j.	Bathing or dressing yourself	❑	❑	❑

4. During the <u>past 4 weeks</u>, have you had any of the following problems with your work or other regular daily activities as a result of your physical health?

		YES	NO
a.	Cut down on the amount of time you spent on work or other activities	❑	❑
b.	Accomplished less than you would like	❑	❑
c.	Were limited in the kind of work or other activities	❑	❑
d.	Had difficulty performing the work or other activities (for example, it took extra effort)	❑	❑

5. During the <u>past 4 weeks</u>, have you had any of the following problems with your work or other regular daily activities as a result of any emotional problems (such as feeling depressed or anxious)?

		YES	NO
a.	Cut down on the amount of time you spent on work or other activities	❑	❑
b.	Accomplished less than you would like	❑	❑
c.	Didn't do work or other activities as carefully as usual	❑	❑

6. During the <u>past 4 weeks</u>, to what extent has your physical health or emotional problems interfered with your normal social activities with family, friends, neighbors, or groups?

❑ Not At All
❑ Slightly
❑ Moderately
❑ Quite a Bit
❑ Extremely

7. How much bodily pain have you had during the <u>past 4 weeks</u>?

❑ None
❑ Very Mild
❑ Mild
❑ Moderate
❑ Severe
❑ Very Severe

8. During the past 4 weeks, how much did pain interfere with your normal work (including both work outside the home and housework)?

❑ Not at All
❑ A Little Bit
❑ Moderately
❑ Quite a Bit
❑ Extremely

9. These questions are about how you feel and how things have been with you during the past 4 weeks. For each question, please give the one answer that comes closest to the way you have been feeling. How much of the time during the <u>past 4 weeks</u>...

	All of the time	Most of the time	A good bit of the time	Some of the time	A little of the time	None of the time
a. Did you feel full of pep?	❑	❑	❑	❑	❑	❑
b. Have you been very nervous?	❑	❑	❑	❑	❑	❑
c. Have you felt calm and peaceful?	❑	❑	❑	❑	❑	❑
d. Did you have a lot of energy?	❑	❑	❑	❑	❑	❑
e. Have you felt down-hearted and blue?	❑	❑	❑	❑	❑	❑
f. Did you feel worn out?	❑	❑	❑	❑	❑	❑
g. Have you been a happy person	❑	❑	❑	❑	❑	❑
h. Did you feel tired?	❑	❑	❑	❑	❑	❑

10. During the <u>past 4 weeks</u>, how much of the time has your physical health or emotional problems interfered with your social activities (like visiting with friends, relatives, etc.)?

❑ All of the time
❑ Most of the time
❑ Some of the time
❑ A little of the time
❑ None of the time

11. How TRUE or FALSE is each of the following statements for you?

		Definitely True	Mostly True	Don't Know	Mostly False	Definitely False
a.	I seem to get sick a little easier than other people	❑	❑	❑	❑	❑
b.	I am as healthy as anybody I know	❑	❑	❑	❑	❑
c.	I expect my health to get worse	❑	❑	❑	❑	❑
d.	My health is excellent	❑	❑	❑	❑	❑

2000 IKDC Subjective Knee Evaluation Form
Patients Part:

Your Full Name_____

Today's Date: _____/_____/_____   Date of Injury: _____/_____/_____
              Day   Month   Year   Day   Month   Year

SYMPTOMS*:
*Grade symptoms at the highest activity level at which you think you could function without significant symptoms, even if you are not actually performing activities at this level.

1. **What is the highest level of activity that you can perform without significant knee pain?**

   ❑ Very strenuous activities like jumping or pivoting as in basketball or soccer
   ❑ Strenuous activities like heavy physical work, skiing or tennis
   ❑ Moderate activities like moderate physical work, running or jogging
   ❑ Light activities like walking, housework or yard work
   ❑ Unable to perform any of the above activities due to knee pain

2. **During the <u>past 4 weeks</u>, or since your injury, how often have you had pain?**

	0	1	2	3	4	5	6	7	8	9	10	
Never	❑	❑	❑	❑	❑	❑	❑	❑	❑	❑	❑	Constant

3. **If you have pain, how severe is it?**

	0	1	2	3	4	5	6	7	8	9	10	
No pain	❑	❑	❑	❑	❑	❑	❑	❑	❑	❑	❑	Worst pain imaginable

4. **During the past 4 weeks, or since your injury, how stiff or swollen was your knee?**
   ❑ Not at all
   ❑ Mildly
   ❑ Moderately
   ❑ Very
   ❑ Extremely

5. **What is the highest level of activity you can perform without significant swelling in your knee?**
   ❑ Very strenuous activities like jumping or pivoting as in basketball or soccer
   ❑ Strenuous activities like heavy physical work, skiing or tennis
   ❑ Moderate activities like moderate physical work, running or jogging
   ❑ Light activities like walking, housework, or yard work
   ❑ Unable to perform any of the above activities due to knee swelling

6. **During the <u>past 4 weeks</u>, or since your injury, did your knee lock or catch?**

   ❑ Yes   ❑ No

7. **What is the highest level of activity you can perform without significant giving way in your knee?**
   ❑ Very strenuous activities like jumping or pivoting as in basketball or soccer
   ❑ Strenuous activities like heavy physical work, skiing or tennis
   ❑ Moderate activities like moderate physical work, running or jogging
   ❑ Light activities like walking, housework or yard work
   ❑ Unable to perform any of the above activities due to giving way of the knee

SPORTS ACTIVITIES:

8. **What is the highest level of activity you can participate in on a regular basis?**

- ❏ Very strenuous activities like jumping or pivoting as in basketball or soccer
- ❏ Strenuous activities like heavy physical work, skiing or tennis
- ❏ Moderate activities like moderate physical work, running or jogging
- ❏ Light activities like walking, housework or yard work
- ❏ Unable to perform any of the above activities due to knee

9. **How does your knee affect your ability to:**

		Not difficult at all	Minimally difficult	Moderately difficult	Extremely difficult	Unable to do
a.	Go up stairs	❏	❏	❏	❏	❏
b.	Go down stairs	❏	❏	❏	❏	❏
c.	Kneel on the front of your knee	❏	❏	❏	❏	❏
d.	Squat	❏	❏	❏	❏	❏
e.	Sit with your knee bent	❏	❏	❏	❏	❏
f.	Rise from a chair	❏	❏	❏	❏	❏
g.	Run straight ahead	❏	❏	❏	❏	❏
h.	Jump and land on your involved leg	❏	❏	❏	❏	❏
i.	Stop and start quickly	❏	❏	❏	❏	❏

FUNCTION:

10. **How would you rate the function of your knee on a scale of 0 to 10 with 10 being normal, excellent function and 0 being the inability to perform any of your usual daily activities which may include sports?**

FUNCTION PRIOR TO YOUR KNEE INJURY:

Cannot perform
daily activities   No limitation

	0	1	2	3	4	5	6	7	8	9	10
	❏	❏	❏	❏	❏	❏	❏	❏	❏	❏	❏

CURRENT FUNCTION OF YOUR KNEE:

Cannot perform
daily activities   No limitation

	0	1	2	3	4	5	6	7	8	9	10
	❏	❏	❏	❏	❏	❏	❏	❏	❏	❏	❏

SCORING INSTRUCTIONS FOR THE 2000 IKDC SUBJECTIVE KNEE EVALUATION FORM

Several methods of scoring the IKDC Subjective Knee Evaluation Form were investigated. The results indicated that summing the scores for each item performed as well as more sophisticated scoring methods.

The responses to each item are scored using an ordinal method such that a score of 1 is given to responses that represent the lowest level of function or highest level of symptoms. For example, item 1, which is related to the highest level of activity without significant pain is scored by assigning a score of 1 to the response "Unable to Perform Any of the Above Activities Due to Knee" and a score of 5 to the response "Very strenuous activities like jumping or pivoting as in basketball or soccer". For item 2, which is related to the frequency of pain over the past 4 weeks, the response "Constant" is assigned a score of 1 and "Never" is assigned a score of 11.

The IKDC Subjective Knee Evaluation Form is scored by summing the scores for the individual items and then transforming the score to a scale that ranges from 0 to 100. **Note:** The response to item 10 "Function Prior to Knee Injury" is not included in the overall score. The steps to score the IKDC Subjective Knee Evaluation Form are as follows:

1. Assign a score to the individual's response for each item, such that lowest score represents the lowest level of function or highest level of symptoms.
2. Calculate the raw score by summing the responses to all items with the exception of the response to item 10 "Function Prior to Your Knee Injury"
3. Transform the raw score to a 0 to 100 scale as follows:

$$\text{IKDC Score} = \left[\frac{\text{Raw Score - Lowest Possible Score}}{\text{Range of Scores}} \right] \times 100$$

Where the lowest possible score is 18 and the range of possible scores is 87. Thus, if the sum of scores for the 18 items is 60, the IKDC Score would be calculated as follows:

$$\text{IKDC Score} = \left[\frac{60 - 18}{87} \right] \times 100$$

$$\text{IKDC Score} = 48.3$$

The transformed score is interpreted as a measure of function such that higher scores represent higher levels of function and lower levels of symptoms. A score of 100 is interpreted to mean no limitation with activities of daily living or sports activities and the absence of symptoms.

The IKDC Subjective Knee Score can still be calculated if there are missing data, as long as there are responses to at least 90% of the items (i.e. responses have been provided for at least 16 items). To calculate the raw IKDC score when there are missing data, substitute the average score of the items that have been answered for the missing item score(s). Once the raw IKDC score has been calculated, it is transformed to the IKDC Subjective Knee Score as described above.

ICRS KNEE HISTORY REGISTRATION – PREVIOUS SURGERY
Surgeons part

Type of surgery: Check all that apply
Meniscal surgery:

Medial meniscal surgery :
Partial resection___ Subtotal resection__
Meniscal suture___
Meniscal Transplant___
Open___Arthroscop___

Lateral Meniscal Surgery
Partial resection___ Subtotal resection__
Meniscal Suture___
Meniscal Transplant___
Open___Arthroscop__

Ligament Surgery:
ACL repair__Intraarticular __ Extraarticular___
PCL-repair__Intraarticular___Extraarticular___
Medial-___Lateral-Collateral-ligament reconstruction___

Type of graft:
Patella-tendon__   Ipsilateral__Contralateral__
Single hamstrings-graft___
2 bundle hamstrings-graft___
4 bundle hamstrings-graft___
Quadriceps-graft___
Allograft___
Other___

Extensor Mechanism surgery:
Patella tendon repair___ Quadriceps-tendon repair___

Patellofemoral surgery:
Soft tissue realignement:
          Medial imbrication___ Lateral release___
Bone realignement:
                    Tibial tubercle transfer:
          Proximal__Distal__Medial__Lateral__Anterior__
                    Trochlear plasty__
                    Patellectomy__

                    Cartilage resurfacing and reconstructive surgery:
                    Debridement (shaving of fibrillated cartile and cartilage flaps)   ____
                    Abrasion arthroplast   ____
                    Microfracture   ____
                    Subchondral drilling   ____
                    Carbon fibre resurfacing   ____
                    Osteochondral allograft   ____
                    Multiple osteochondral autologous grafts   ____
                    Periosteal resurfacing   ____
                    Perichondral resurfacing   ____
                    Autologous chondrocyte implantation + periosteum   ____
                    Autologous chondrocyte implantation with membrane   ____
                    Other type of technique: _____   ____

Surgeons part

Osteotomy: Tibia____Femur____ Varus____Valgus_____

Imaging techniques:

Plain x-rays:_____ Varus-angle_____Valgus-angle_____

CT____ CT-arthrography____ MRI____ Scintigraphy_____

Findings:

Articular cartilage appearance:_____

_____

Bone:_____ _____

_____

Ligaments:_____ _____

_____

Menisci:_____ _____

_____

2000 IKDC KNEE Examination Form
Surgeons part

Patient Name :_____ Date of Birth: ____/_____/_____
                                                                 Day   Month   Year

Gender: ? F   ? M   Age :_____ Date of Examination:____/_____/_____
                                                                   Day   Month   Year

Generalized Laxity:	?tight	?normal	?lax
Alignment:	?obvious varus	?normal	?obvious valgus
Patella Position:	?obvious baja	?normal	?obvious alta
Patella Subluxation/Dislocation:	?centered	?subluxable	?subluxed	?dislocated

Range of Motion (Ext/Flex):   Index Side: passive_____/_____/_____   active_____/_____/_____
                                  Opposite Side: passive_____/_____/_____   active_____/_____/_____

SEVEN GROUPS	FOUR GRADES				*Group Grade			
	A Normal	B Nearly Normal	C Abnormal	D Severely Abnormal	A	B	C	D
1. Effusion	? None	? Mild	? Moderate	? Severe	?	?	?	?
2. Passive Motion Deficit								
∆Lack of extension	? <3°	? 3 to 5°	? 6 to 10°	? >10°				
∆Lack of flexion	? 0 to 5°	? 6 to 15°	? 16 to 25°	? >25°	?	?	?	?
3. Ligament Examination								
(manual, instrumented, x-ray)								
∆Lachman (25° flex) (134N)	? -1 to 2mm	? 3 to 5mm(1⁺) ? <-1 to –3	? 6 to 10mm(2⁺) ? <-3 stiff	? >10mm(3⁺)				
∆Lachman (25° flex) manual max	? -1 to 2mm	? 3 to 5mm	? 6 to 10mm	? >10mm				
Anterior endpoint:	? firm		? soft					
∆Total AP Translation (25° flex)	? 0 to 2mm	? 3 to 5mm	? 6 to 10mm	? >10mm				
∆Total AP Translation (70° flex)	? 0 to 2mm	? 3 to 5mm	? 6 to 10mm	? >10mm				
∆Posterior Drawer Test (70° flex)	? 0 to 2mm	? 3 to 5mm	? 6 to 10mm	? >10mm				
∆Med Joint Opening (20° flex/valgus rot)	? 0 to 2mm	? 3 to 5mm	? 6 to 10mm	?>10mm				
∆Lat Joint Opening (20° flex/varus rot)	? 0 to 2mm	? 3 to 5mm	? 6 to 10mm	? >10mm				
∆External Rotation Test (30° flex prone)	? <5°	? 6 to 10°	? 11 to 19°	? >20°				
∆External Rotation Test (90° flex prone)	? <5°	? 6 to 10°	? 11 to 19°	? >20°				
∆Pivot Shift	? equal	? +glide	? ++(clunk)	? +++(gross)				
∆Reverse Pivot Shift	? equal	? glide	? gross	? marked				
					?	?	?	?
4. Compartment Findings		crepitation with						
∆Crepitus Ant. Compartment	? none	? moderate	? mild pain	? >mild pain				
∆Crepitus Med. Compartment	? none	? moderate	? mild pain	? >mild pain				
∆Crepitus Lat. Compartment	? none	? moderate	? mild pain	? >mild pain				
5. Harvest Site Pathology	? none	? mild	? moderate	? severe				
6. X-ray Findings								
Med. Joint Space	? none	? mild	? moderate	? severe				
Lat. Joint Space	? none	? mild	? moderate	? severe				
Patellofemoral	? none	? mild	? moderate	?severe				
Ant. Joint Space (sagittal)	? none	? mild	? moderate	? severe				
Post. Joint Space (sagittal)	? none	? mild	? moderate	? severe				
7. Functional Test								
One Leg Hop (% of opposite side)	? ≥90%	? 89 to 76%	? 75 to 50%	? <50%				
**Final Evaluation					?	?	?	?

*   Group grade: The lowest grade within a group determines the group grade
** Final evaluation: the worst group grade determines the final evaluation for acute and subacute patients. For chronic patients compare preoperative and postoperative evaluations. In a final evaluation only the first 3 groups are evaluated but all groups must be documented. ∆ Difference in involved knee compared to normal or what is assumed to be normal.

IKDC COMMITTEE AOSSM: Anderson, A., Bergfeld, J., Boland, A. Dye, S., Feagin, J., Harner, C. Mohtadi, N. Richmond, J. Shelbourne, D., Terry, G. ESSKA: Staubli, H., Hefti, F., Hoher, J., Jacob, R., Mueller, W., Neyret, P.   APOSSM: Chan, K., Kurosaka, M.

CARTILAGE REPAIR ASSESSMENT

Criteria	Points	
Degree of Defect Repair I **Protocol A** [1]	* In level with surrounding cartilage * 75% repair of defect depth * 50% repair of defect depth * 25% repair of defect depth * 0% repair of defect depth	4 3 2 1 0
I **Protocol B** [2]	* 100% survival of initially grafted surface * 75% survival of initially grafted surface * 50% survival of initially grafted surface * 25% survival of initially grafted surface * 0% (plugs are lost or broken)	4 3 2 1 0
II **Integration to Border zone**	* Complete integration with surrounding cartilage * Demarcating border < 1mm * 3/4 of graft integrated, 1/4 with a notable border >1mm width * 1/2 of graft integrated with surrounding cartilage, 1/2 with a notable border > 1mm * From no contact to 1/4 of graft integrated with surrounding cartilage	4 3 2 1 0
III **Macroscopic Appearance**	* Intact smooth surface * Fibrillated surface * Small, scattered fissures or cracs * Several, small or few but large fissures * Total degeneration of grafted area	4 3 2 1 0
Overall Repair Assessment	Grade I normal Grade II nearly normal Grade III abnormal Grade IV severely abnormal	12 P 11-8 P 7-4 P 3-1 P

Cartilage Biopsy   Location _____

(1) **Protocol A:**	(2) **Protocol B:**
autologous chondrocyte implantation (ACI); periosteal or perichondrial transplantation; subchondral drilling; microfracturing; carbon fibre implants; others:	Mosaicplasty; OAT; osteochondral allografts; others:

INSTRUCTIONS FOR THE 2000 IKDC KNEE EXAMINATION FORM

The Knee Examination Form contains items that fall into one of seven measurement domains. However, only the first three of these domains are graded. The seven domains assessed by the Knee Examination Form are:

1. *Effusion*
    An effusion is assessed by ballotting the knee. A fluid wave (less than 25 cc) is graded mild, easily ballotteable fluid – moderate (25-60 cc), and a tense knee secondary to effusion (greater than 60 cc) is rated severe.

2. *Passive Motion Deficit*
    Passive range of motion is measured with a gonimeter and recorded on the form for the index side and opposite or normal side. Record values for zero point/hyperextension/flexion (e.g. 10 degrees of hyperextension, 150 degrees of flexion = 10/0/150; 10 degrees of flexion to 150 degrees of flexion = 0/10/150). Extension is compared to that of the normal knee.

3. *Ligament Examination*
    The Lachman test, total AP translation at 70 degrees, and medial and lateral joint opening may be assessed with manual, instrumented or stress x-ray examination. Only one should be graded, preferably a "measured displacement". A force of 134 N (30 lbs) and the maximum manual are recorded in instrumented examination of both knees. Only the measured displacement at the standard force of 134 N is used for grading. The numerical values for the side to side difference are rounded off, and the appropriate box is marked.

    The end point is assessed in the Lachman test. The end point affects the grading when the index knee has 3-5 mm more anterior laxity than the normal knee. In this case, a soft end point results in an abnormal grade rather than a nearly normal grade.

    The 70-degree posterior sag is estimated by comparing the profile of the injured knee to the normal knee and palpating the medial femoral tibia step off. It may be confirmed by noting that contraction of the quadriceps pulls the tibia interiorly.

    The external rotation tests are performed with the patient prone and the knee flexed 30° and 70°.
    Equal external rotational torque is applied to both feet and the degree of external rotation is recorded.

    The pivot shift and reverse pivot shift are performed with the patient supine, with the hip in 10-20 degrees of abduction and the tibia in neutral rotation using either the Losee, Noyes, or Jakob techniques. The greatest subluxation, compared to the normal knee, should be recorded.

4. *Compartment Findings*
    Patellofemoral crepitation is elicited by extension against slight resistance. Medial and lateral compartment crepitation is elicited by extending the knee from a flexed position with a varus stress and then a valgus stress (i.e., McMurray test). Grading is based on intensity and pain.

5. *Harvest Site Pathology*
    Note tenderness, irritation or numbness at the autograft harvest site.

6. *X-ray Findings*
    A bilateral, double leg PA weightbearing roentgenogram at 35-45 degrees of flexion (tunnel view) is used to evaluate narrowing of the medial and lateral joint spaces. The Merchant view at 45 degrees is used to document patellofemoral narrowing. A mild grade indicates minimal changes (i.e., small osteophytes, slight sclerosis or flattening of the femoral condyle) and narrowing of the joint space which is just detectable. A moderate grade may have those changes and joint space narrowing (e.g., a joint space of 2-4 mm side or up to 50% joint space narrowing). Severe changes include a joint space of less than 2 mm or greater than 50% joint space narrowing.

7. *Functional Test*
    The patient is asked to perform a one leg hop for distance on the index and normal side. Three trials for each leg are recorded and averaged. A ratio of the index to normal knee is calculated.

ICRS Grade 0 - Normal

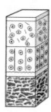

ICRS Grade 1 – Nearly Normal
Superficial lesions. Soft indentation (A) and/or superficial fissures and cracks (B)

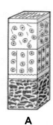 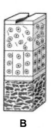

A   B

ICRS Grade 2 – Abnormal
Lesions extending down to <50% of cartilage depth

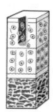

ICRS Grade 3 – Severely Abnormal
Cartilage defects extending down >50% of cartilage depth (A) as well as down to calcified layer (B) and down to but not through the subchondral bone (C). Blisters are included in this Grade (D)

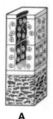 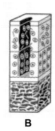 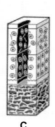 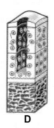

A   B   C   D

ICRS Grade 4 – Severely Abnormal

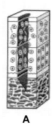 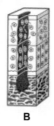

A   B

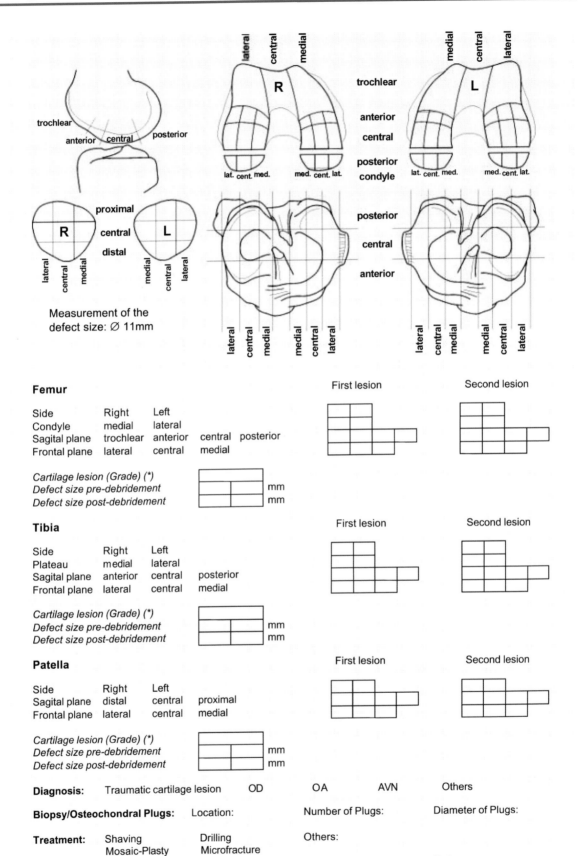

Measurement of the
defect size: Ø 11mm

Femur

Side	Right	Left		
Condyle	medial	lateral		
Sagital plane	trochlear	anterior	central	posterior
Frontal plane	lateral	central	medial	

First lesion   Second lesion

Cartilage lesion (Grade) (*)
Defect size pre-debridement _____ mm
Defect size post-debridement _____ mm

Tibia

Side	Right	Left	
Plateau	medial	lateral	
Sagital plane	anterior	central	posterior
Frontal plane	lateral	central	medial

First lesion   Second lesion

Cartilage lesion (Grade) (*)
Defect size pre-debridement _____ mm
Defect size post-debridement _____ mm

Patella

Side	Right	Left	
Sagital plane	distal	central	proximal
Frontal plane	lateral	central	medial

First lesion   Second lesion

Cartilage lesion (Grade) (*)
Defect size pre-debridement _____ mm
Defect size post-debridement _____ mm

Diagnosis: Traumatic cartilage lesion   OD   OA   AVN   Others

Biopsy/Osteochondral Plugs: Location: Number of Plugs: Diameter of Plugs:

Treatment: Shaving   Drilling   Others:
                Mosaic-Plasty   Microfracture
                Autologous Chondrocyte Implantation (ACI)   **Notes:**

ICRS Classification of OCD-Lesions (Osteochondritis-Dissecans)

ICRS OCD I

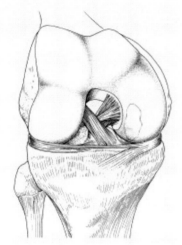

Stable, continuity: Softened area covered by intact cartilage.

ICRS OCD II

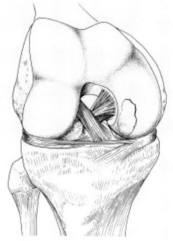

Partial discontinuity, stable on probing

ICRS OCD III

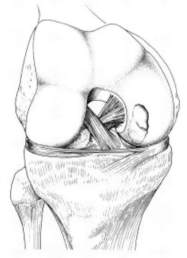

Complete discontinuity, "dead in situ", not dislocated.

ICRS OCD IV

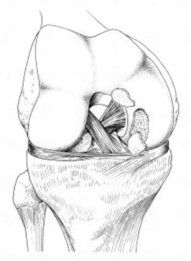

Dislocated fragment, loose within the bed or empty defect.> 10mm in depth is B-subgroup

KOOS KNEE SURVEY

Todays date: _____/_____/_____ Date of birth: _____/_____/_____

Name: _____

INSTRUCTIONS: This survey asks for your view about your knee. This information will help us keep track of how you feel about your knee and how well you are able to do your usual activities.
Answer every question by ticking the appropriate box, only <u>one</u> box for each question. If you are unsure about how to answer a question, please give the best answer you can.

Symptoms
These questions should be answered thinking of your knee symptoms during the **last week**.

S1. Do you have swelling in your knee?

Never	Rarely	Sometimes	Often	Always
☐	☐	☐	☐	☐

S2. Do you feel grinding, hear clicking or any other type of noise when your knee moves?

Never	Rarely	Sometimes	Often	Always
☐	☐	☐	☐	☐

S3. Does your knee catch or hang up when moving?

Never	Rarely	Sometimes	Often	Always
☐	☐	☐	☐	☐

S4. Can you straighten your knee fully?

Always	Often	Sometimes	Rarely	Never
☐	☐	☐	☐	☐

S5. Can you bend your knee fully?

Always	Often	Sometimes	Rarely	Never
☐	☐	☐	☐	☐

Stiffness
The following questions concern the amount of joint stiffness you have experienced during the **last week** in your knee. Stiffness is a sensation of restriction or slowness in the ease with which you move your knee joint.

S6. How severe is your knee joint stiffness after first wakening in the morning?

None	Mild	Moderate	Severe	Extreme
☐	☐	☐	☐	☐

S7. How severe is your knee stiffness after sitting, lying or resting **later in the day**?

None	Mild	Moderate	Severe	Extreme
☐	☐	☐	☐	☐

Pain

P1. How often do you experience knee pain?

Never	Monthly	Weekly	Daily	Always
☐	☐	☐	☐	☐

What amount of knee pain have you experienced the **last week** during the following activities?

P2. Twisting/pivoting on your knee

None	Mild	Moderate	Severe	Extreme
☐	☐	☐	☐	☐

P3. Straightening knee fully

None	Mild	Moderate	Severe	Extreme
☐	☐	☐	☐	☐

P4. Bending knee fully

None	Mild	Moderate	Severe	Extreme
☐	☐	☐	☐	☐

P5. Walking on flat surface

None	Mild	Moderate	Severe	Extreme
☐	☐	☐	☐	☐

P6. Going up or down stairs

None	Mild	Moderate	Severe	Extreme
☐	☐	☐	☐	☐

P7. At night while in bed

None	Mild	Moderate	Severe	Extreme
☐	☐	☐	☐	☐

P8. Sitting or lying

None	Mild	Moderate	Severe	Extreme
☐	☐	☐	☐	☐

P9. Standing upright

None	Mild	Moderate	Severe	Extreme
☐	☐	☐	☐	☐

Function, daily living

The following questions concern your physical function. By this we mean your ability to move around and to look after yourself. For each of the following activities please indicate the degree of difficulty you have experienced in the **last week** due to your knee.

A1. Descending stairs

None	Mild	Moderate	Severe	Extreme
☐	☐	☐	☐	☐

A2. Ascending stairs

None	Mild	Moderate	Severe	Extreme
☐	☐	☐	☐	☐

For each of the following activities please indicate the degree of difficulty you have experienced in the **last week** due to your knee.

A3. Rising from sitting

None	Mild	Moderate	Severe	Extreme
☐	☐	☐	☐	☐

A4. Standing

None	Mild	Moderate	Severe	Extreme
☐	☐	☐	☐	☐

A5. Bending to floor/pick up an object

None	Mild	Moderate	Severe	Extreme
☐	☐	☐	☐	☐

A6. Walking on flat surface

None	Mild	Moderate	Severe	Extreme
☐	☐	☐	☐	☐

A7. Getting in/out of car

None	Mild	Moderate	Severe	Extreme
☐	☐	☐	☐	☐

A8. Going shopping

None	Mild	Moderate	Severe	Extreme
☐	☐	☐	☐	☐

A9. Putting on socks/stockings

None	Mild	Moderate	Severe	Extreme
☐	☐	☐	☐	☐

A10. Rising from bed

None	Mild	Moderate	Severe	Extreme
☐	☐	☐	☐	☐

A11. Taking off socks/stockings

None	Mild	Moderate	Severe	Extreme
☐	☐	☐	☐	☐

A12. Lying in bed (turning over, maintaining knee position)

None	Mild	Moderate	Severe	Extreme
☐	☐	☐	☐	☐

A13. Getting in/out of bath

None	Mild	Moderate	Severe	Extreme
☐	☐	☐	☐	☐

A14. Sitting

None	Mild	Moderate	Severe	Extreme
☐	☐	☐	☐	☐

A15. Getting on/off toilet

None	Mild	Moderate	Severe	Extreme
☐	☐	☐	☐	☐

For each of the following activities please indicate the degree of difficulty you have experienced in the **last week** due to your knee.

A16. Heavy domestic duties (moving heavy boxes, scrubbing floors, etc)

None	Mild	Moderate	Severe	Extreme
☐	☐	☐	☐	☐

A17. Light domestic duties (cooking, dusting, etc)

None	Mild	Moderate	Severe	Extreme
☐	☐	☐	☐	☐

Function, sports and recreational activities

The following questions concern your physical function when being active on a higher level. The questions should be answered thinking of what degree of difficulty you have experienced during the **last week** due to your knee.

SP1. Squatting

None	Mild	Moderate	Severe	Extreme
☐	☐	☐	☐	☐

SP2. Running

None	Mild	Moderate	Severe	Extreme
☐	☐	☐	☐	☐

SP3. Jumping

None	Mild	Moderate	Severe	Extreme
☐	☐	☐	☐	☐

SP4. Twisting/pivoting on your injured knee

None	Mild	Moderate	Severe	Extreme
☐	☐	☐	☐	☐

SP5. Kneeling

None	Mild	Moderate	Severe	Extreme
☐	☐	☐	☐	☐

Quality of Life

Q1. How often are you aware of your knee problem?

Never	Monthly	Weekly	Daily	Constantly
☐	☐	☐	☐	☐

Q2. Have you modified your life style to avoid potentially damaging activities to your knee?

Not at all	Mildly	Moderatly	Severely	Totally
☐	☐	☐	☐	☐

Q3. How much are you troubled with lack of confidence in your knee?

Not at all	Mildly	Moderately	Severely	Extremely
☐	☐	☐	☐	☐

Q4. In general, how much difficulty do you have with your knee?

None	Mild	Moderate	Severe	Extreme
☐	☐	☐	☐	☐

Thank you very much for completing all the questions in this questionnaire.

A User's Guide to:
Knee injury and Osteoarthritis Outcome Score KOOS

KOOS is developed as an instrument to assess the patients opinion about their knee and associated problems.

KOOS is intended to be used for knee injury that can result in post traumatic osteoarthritis (OA); i.e. ACL (anterior cruciate ligament) injury, meniscus injury, chondral injury, etc.

KOOS is meant to be used over short and long time intervals; to assess changes from week to week induced by treatment (medication, operation, physical therapy) or over years due to the primary injury or post traumatic OA.

KOOS can be used to assess groups and to monitor individuals.

KOOS content validity was ensured through literature search, a pilot study and an expert panel (US and Sweden); patients, orthopedic surgeons and physical therapists.

KOOS consists of 5 subscales; **Pain**, other **Symptoms**, **Function in daily living (ADL)**, **Function in sport and recreation (Sport/Rec)** and **knee related Quality of life QOL**. The last week is taken into consideration when answering the questions. Standardized answer options are given (5 Likert boxes) and each question gets a score from 0 to 4. A normalized score (100 indicating no symptoms and 0 indicating extreme symptoms) is calculated *for each subscale.* The result can be plotted as an outcome profile.

KOOS is patient-administered, the format is user friendly, and takes about 10 minutes to fill out.

KOOS is self-explanatory and can be administered in the waiting room or used as a mailed survey.

KOOS has been used in patients 14-78 years old.

KOOS reference values from a group of 50 subjects (mean 53 years, 37-79) with no previous and no current clinical signs of injury to the ACL or menisci and no radiographic signs of OA has been established [1].

KOOS has high test-retest reproducibility (ICC >0.75).

KOOS includes WOMAC Osteoarthritis Index LK 3.0 [2] in its complete and original format (with permission), and WOMAC scores can be calculated. WOMAC is valid for elderly subjects with knee OA.

KOOS construct validity has been determined in comparison with SF-36 [3, 4] and expected correlations were found [5-7]. Moderates to high correlations were found when comparing to the Lysholm knee scoring scale [6].

KOOS subscales "Sport and Recreation function" and "Quality of Life" were more sensitive and discriminative than the WOMAC subscales "Pain", "Stiffness", and "Function" when studied in subjects meniscectomized 21 years ago and with definite radiographic signs of OA (mean 57 years, 38-76) compared to age- and gendermatched controls [8].

KOOS responsiveness has been determined in three separate studies. Significant improvement was found after reconstruction of the ACL [7], after physical therapy [7], three months after arthroscopic partial meniscectomy [6] and 6 months after total knee replacement [5]. High effect sizes (mean score change/preoperative SD) were found, indicating fewer subjects needed to yield statistically significant differences.

KOOS validation work is ongoing. KOOS is currently being used in several clinical studies involving patients with meniscus injury, ACL-injury, cartilage injury, and post-traumatic osteoarthritis (for current update search PubMed using "KOOS + knee"). Several methodological papers regarding the KOOS have been published [5-8].

KOOS is currently available in the following versions, American-English, Swedish, Danish, and German. Unvalidated versions in Italian and Russian are available. The validation work of French and Spanish versions are ongoing.

KOOS information can be required from:

Ewa Roos PT PhD, Department of Orthopedics, Lund University Hospital, S-221 85 Lund, Sweden.
Fax: int+46(46) 13 07 32 E-mail: Ewa.Roos@ort.lu.se

REFERENCES

1. EM Roos, M Klassbo, LS Lohmander: **WOMAC osteoarthritis index. Reliability, validity, and responsiveness in patients with arthroscopically assessed osteoarthritis. Western Ontario and MacMaster Universities**. *Scand J Rheumatol* 1999, **28**:210-5.

2. N Bellamy, WW Buchanan, CH Goldsmith, J Campbell, LW Stitt: **Validation study of WOMAC: a health status instrument for measuring clinically important patient relevant outcomes to antirheumatic drug therapy in patients with osteoarthritis of the hip or knee**. *J Rheumatol* 1988, **15**:1833-40.

3. JE Ware, Jr., CD Sherbourne: **The MOS 36-item short-form health survey (SF-36). I. Conceptual framework and item selection**. *Med Care* 1992, **30**:473-83.

4. JE Ware, Jr., K Snow, M Kosinski, B Gandek: **SF-36 Health Survey Manual and Interpretation Guide**. Boston, MA: The Health Institute, New England Medical Center; 1993.

5. E Roos, S Toksvig-Larsen: **Knee injury and Osteoarthritis Outcome Score (KOOS) -validation and comparison to the WOMAC in total knee replacement**. *Health and Quality of Life Outcomes* 2003, **1**.

6. EM Roos, HP Roos, C Ekdahl, LS Lohmander: **Knee injury and Osteoarthritis Outcome Score (KOOS)--validation of a Swedish version**. *Scand J Med Sci Sports* 1998, **8**:439-48.

7. EM Roos, HP Roos, LS Lohmander, C Ekdahl, BD Beynnon: **Knee Injury and Osteoarthritis Outcome Score (KOOS)--development of a self-administered outcome measure**. *J Orthop Sports Phys Ther* 1998, **28**:88-96.

8. EM Roos, HP Roos, LS Lohmander: **WOMAC Osteoarthritis Index-- additional dimensions for use in subjects with post-traumatic osteoarthritis of the knee. Western Ontario and MacMaster Universities**. *Osteoarthritis Cartilage* 1999, **7**:216-21.

KOOS *Reference data*
- ACL-reconstruction, meniscectomy, and post-traumatic OA

KOOS has been used in studies of anterior cruciate ligament (ACL) injury, meniscus injury, and post-traumatic osteoarthritis (OA). KOOS scores from three of these studies are given to enable KOOS-users to get familiar with the score. **To make scientific comparisons, use to the original articles referred to in each section!** The data is visualized in graphs. The mean scores for all five subscales are given and connected with a line which gives a **KOOS Profile.** 0 indicates extreme problems and 100 indicate no problems.

ACL data
(From: Roos E, Roos H, Lohmander LS, Ekdahl C, Beynnon B. Knee injury and Osteoarthritis Outcome Score (KOOS) - Development of a self-administered outcome measure. The Journal of Orthopaedic and Sports Physical Therapy 78(2)88-96, 1998.)
In figure 1 data is given for 21 American subjects (9 males and 12 females) with ACL injury about to undergo reconstruction. Ten of the subjects had a combined meniscus injury. Their mean age was 32 (range 18 to 46). The majority had sustained their knee injury less than 6 months prior to operation. Ten subjects were competing in sports and nine were recreational athletes.

Interpretation: The Sport/Rec and Quality of Life subscales are the most sensitive subscales pre-operatively and changes the most post-operatively. ACL-injury affect daily life (ADL) little, and there is little room for improvement in this subscale. The Symptom score of 91 one year after reconstruction is primarily due to lack of full knee flexion. As known from clinical experience, pain is not a major symptom of ACL injury. The score of 80 pre-operatively can be due to ten subjects having an associated meniscus injury. When considering Pain, Symptoms, ADL and Sport/Rec the subjects can be considered having very little problems one year after surgery. They are mentally still aware of their knee though, as seen by a score of 75 in the subscale Quality of Life.

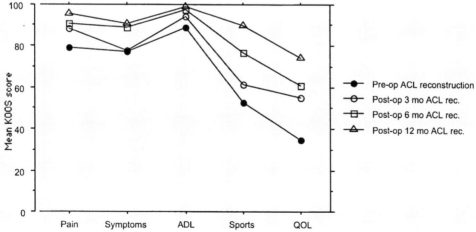

Figure 1. ACL reconstruction

Meniscus data

(From: Roos E, Roos H, Ekdahl C, Lohmander LS. Knee injury and Osteoarthritis Outcome Score (KOOS) - validation of a Swedish version. Scandinavian Journal of Medicine and Science in Sports: 8, 439-448, 1998.)

In figure 2, data from 95 Swedish subjects (33 females) having an arthroscopic partial meniscectomy is reported. Their mean age was 42, ranging from 14 to 75. Mean duration of symptoms was one year, ranging from three months to more than 10 years. Approximately 50% had isolated tears, 25% had an associated ACL-injury, and 25% had associated cartilage damage.

Interpretation: A meniscus injury is associated with pain and symptoms such as limited range of motion, swelling, noise and catching. Pre-operatively, low scores are seen fin all scales. The KOOS profile 3 months post-operatively is comparable to the pre-operative profile of ACL reconstruction, with the exception of Quality of Life. It is surprising to see that the subjects still have significant problems three months after a meniscectomy. As previously seen in the ACL-group the subjects report more problems with Sport and Recreation Function and Quality of Life than with the other subscales. This is interesting since the other subscales (Pain, Symptoms and ADL) are the ones usually assessed clinically. When taking associated injuries into consideration, cartilage changes seen at arthroscopy was associated with generally lower scores, while an associated ACL injury was associated with generally higher scores. The pre- and post-operative profiles for isolated meniscus were very similar to the profiles in figure 2.

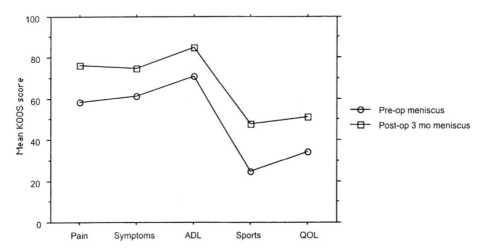

Figure 2. Meniscus data

OA data

(From: Roos E, Roos H, Lohmander LS. WOMAC Osteoarthritis Index - additional dimensions for use in post-traumatic osteoarthritis of the knee. Osteoarthritis and Cartilage: 7(3),216-221, 1999.)

A cohort operated on with open meniscectomy 21 years ago was asked to participate in a follow-up study. In figure 3 data from 41 subjects with radiological OA (defined as Kellgren and Lawrence ≥2) is compared to 50 subjects without radiographic OA from an age and sex-matched control group without known injury to the menisci or ACL, or radiographic OA. Mean age of the OA group was 57 years (range 38-76).

Interpretation: Statistical differences between the groups were found for all five subscales. However the Sport and Recreation and Quality of Life subscales are more discriminative than the other subscales. Symptom is the subscale scoring the lowest in the control group, primarily due to reported grinding, clicking or other noise from the knee. The profile of the post-meniscectomy OA group operated on 21 years ago can roughly be compared to the profile of the post-meniscectomy group operated on 3 months ago. It must be remembered that the subjects in the 21 year post-meniscectomy group were not patients seeking medical care for their knee problems but taking part in a follow-up study. The only criterion used to define OA was positive radiography (Kellgren and Lawrence ≥2).

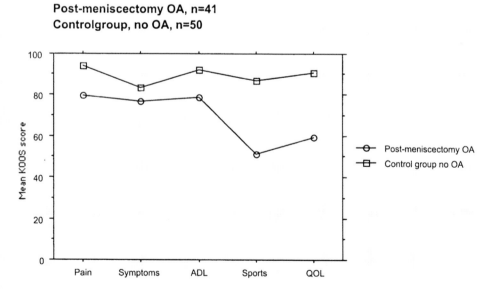

Figure 3. Post-traumatic OA versus an age and sex-matched control group without OA.

KOOS *Manual scoring sheet*

Instructions:
Assign the following scores to the boxes!

None	Mild	Moderate	Severe	Extreme
☐	☐	☐	☐	☐
0	1	2	3	4

Missing data. If a mark is placed outside a box, the closest box is chosen. If two boxes are marked, that which indicated the more severe problems is chosen. Missing data are treated as such; one or two missing values are substituted with the average value for that subscale. If more than two items are omitted, the response is considered invalid and no subscale score is calculated.

Sum up the total score of each subscale and divide by the possible maximum score for the scale. Traditionally in orthopedics, 100 indicates no problems and 0 indicates extreme problems. The normalized score is transformed to meet this standard. Please use the formulas provided for each subscale!

1. PAIN $\qquad 100 - \dfrac{\text{Total score P1-P9 x 100}}{36} = 100 - \dfrac{\rule{2cm}{0.4pt}}{36} = \rule{2cm}{0.4pt}$

2. SYMPTOMS $\qquad 100 - \dfrac{\text{Total score S1-S7 x 100}}{28} = 100 - \dfrac{\rule{2cm}{0.4pt}}{28} = \rule{2cm}{0.4pt}$

3. ADL $\qquad 100 - \dfrac{\text{Total score A1-A17 x 100}}{68} = 100 - \dfrac{\rule{2cm}{0.4pt}}{68} = \rule{2cm}{0.4pt}$

4. SPORT&REC $\qquad 100 - \dfrac{\text{Total score SP1-SP5 x 100}}{20} = 100 - \dfrac{\rule{2cm}{0.4pt}}{20} = \rule{2cm}{0.4pt}$

5. QOL $\qquad 100 - \dfrac{\text{Total score Q1-Q4 x 100}}{16} = 100 - \dfrac{\rule{2cm}{0.4pt}}{16} = \rule{2cm}{0.4pt}$

WOMAC *How to score from the KOOS*

Assign scores from 0 to 4 to the boxes as shown above. To get original WOMAC scores sum the item scores for each subscale. If you prefer percentage scores in accordance with the KOOS, use the formula provided below to convert the original WOMAC scores.

$$\text{Transformed scale} = 100 - \frac{\text{actual raw score} \times 100}{\text{Possible raw score range}}$$

WOMAC subscores	Original score = sum of the following items	Possible raw score range
Pain	P5-P9	20
Stiffness	S6-S7	8
Function	A1-A17	68

KOOS *Profile*

To visualize differences in the five different KOOS subscores and change between different administrations of the KOOS (e.g. pre-treatment to post-treatment), KOOS Profiles can be plotted.

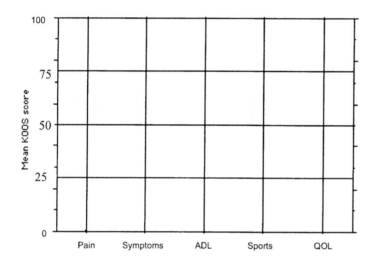

Legend

Symbol/color	Description (pre-treatment, post-treatment etc)	Date

Name: _____

Modified Cincinnati Score (Cartilage Repair Registry)

CARTICEL^SM Service Registry

Registry Number: _____   Patient Initials

☐☐☐

TO BE COMPLETED BY CLINICAL STAFF

BIOPSY HARVESTING VISIT

3/12/96

Patient Demographics

Date of birth:

☐☐☐☐☐☐

Height:

☐☐☐ cm.

Gender:
☐ female   ☐ male

Weight:

☐☐☐ kg.

Orthopedic Surgical History

Check the number of surgical procedures in the last 5 years.

LEFT KNEE	**RIGHT KNEE**
Diagnostic arthroscopy: ☐0 ☐1 ☐2 ☐≥3	**Diagnostic arthroscopy:** ☐0 ☐1 ☐2 ☐≥3
Debridement/Lavage: ☐0 ☐1 ☐2 ☐≥3	**Debridement/Lavage:** ☐0 ☐1 ☐2 ☐≥3
Abrasion/Drilling/Microfracture: ☐0 ☐1 ☐2 ☐≥3	**Abrasion/Drilling/Microfracture:** ☐0 ☐1 ☐2 ☐≥3
Meniscus repair/Meniscectomy: ☐0 ☐1 ☐2 ☐≥3 ☐ medial ☐ lateral ☐ both	**Meniscus repair/Meniscectomy:** ☐0 ☐1 ☐2 ☐≥3 ☐ medial ☐ lateral ☐ both
Ligament repair/Reconstruction: ☐0 ☐1 ☐2 ☐≥3 *(check all that apply)* ☐ACL ☐MCL ☐PCL ☐LCL	**Ligament repair/Reconstruction:** ☐0 ☐1 ☐2 ☐≥3 *(check all that apply)* ☐ACL ☐MCL ☐PCL ☐LCL
Tibial osteotomy: ☐0 ☐1 ☐2 ☐≥3	**Tibial osteotomy:** ☐0 ☐1 ☐2 ☐≥3
Other, specify: _____ ☐0 ☐1 ☐2 ☐≥3	**Other, specify:** _____ ☐0 ☐1 ☐2 ☐≥3

Etiology and Onset

Etiology:
☐ sports   ☐ fall   ☐ motor vehicle accident
☐ daily activities   ☐ unknown

Injury date:
☐☐ – ☐☐

Onset:
☐ acute   ☐ gradual

Symptom onset:
☐☐ – ☐☐

Clinician's Evaluation

Rate the patient according to the following scale.

☐1 ☐2 ☐3 ☐4 ☐5 ☐6 ☐7 ☐8 ☐9 ☐10
poor   fair   good   very good   excellent

Poor (2) .... Patient has significant limitations in daily activities.
Fair (4) .... Patient has moderate limitations that affect daily activities, no sports possible.
Good (6) .... Patient has some limitations with sports but can participate by compensating.
Very good (8) . Patient has only a few limitations with sports.
Excellent (10) Patient is able to do whatever they wish (any sport) with no problems.

Pre Operative Diagnosis

Pre operative diagnosis: _____

Cartilage Grading Scale

Grade the cartilage of the defect area.
☐ **Grade I**   Softening and swelling.
☐ **Grade II**   Fragmentation and fissuring, < 1/2 inch (= 1.27 cm) in diameter.
☐ **Grade III** Fragmentation and fissuring, > 1/2 inch (= 1.27 cm) in diameter.
☐ **Grade IV**   Erosion of cartilage down to the bone.

Type of Defects

☐ focal acute defects   ☐ focal degenerative defects

Biopsy Harvesting Procedure

Date of biopsy:

☐☐☐☐☐

Biopsy taken from:
☐ left knee   ☐ right knee
☐ other, specify: _____

Size of defect:	**Defect #1**	**Defect #2**	**Defect #3**
Length (mm):	☐☐	☐☐	☐☐
Width (mm):	☐☐	☐☐	☐☐

Biopsy site:
☐ medial femoral condyle   ☐ intercondylar notch
☐ lateral femoral condyle   ☐ other, specify: _____

Concurrent Procedures

Debridement/Lavage:
☐ No   ☐ Yes

Meniscus repair/Meniscectomy: *(check only one)*
☐ No   ☐ Yes   ☐ medial   ☐ lateral   ☐ both

Ligament repair/Reconstruction: *(check all that apply)*
☐ No   ☐ Yes   ☐ ACL ☐ MCL ☐ PCL ☐ LCL

Fragment Reattachment/Removal:
☐ No   ☐ Yes

Other:
☐ No   ☐ Yes, specify: _____

Knee Examination

Conduct on BOTH knees. NOT under anaesthesia.

LEFT KNEE	**RIGHT KNEE**
Extension: ☐☐ ° **Flexion:** ☐☐☐ °	**Extension:** ☐☐ ° **Flexion:** ☐☐☐ °
Alignment: ☐ extreme varus < 0° ☐ varus 0° to < 5° ☐ normal 5° to < 10° ☐ valgus 10° to < 15° ☐ extreme valgus ≥ 15°	**Alignment:** ☐ extreme varus < 0° ☐ varus 0° to < 5° ☐ normal 5° to < 10° ☐ valgus 10° to < 15° ☐ extreme valgus ≥ 15°
Anteroposterior stability (mm): ☐ < 5 ☐ 5 to < 10 ☐ ≥10	**Anteroposterior stability (mm):** ☐ < 5 ☐ 5 to < 10 ☐ ≥10
Mediolateral stability: ☐ < 5° ☐ 5° to < 10° ☐ 10° to < 15° ☐ ≥ 15°	**Mediolateral stability:** ☐ < 5° ☐ 5° to < 10° ☐ 10° to < 15° ☐ ≥ 15°
Crepitus: ☐ none ☐ mild ☐ moderate ☐ severe	**Crepitus:** ☐ none ☐ mild ☐ moderate ☐ severe
Effusion: ☐ none ☐ mild ☐ moderate ☐ severe	**Effusion:** ☐ none ☐ mild ☐ moderate ☐ severe
Joint line pain: ☐ none ☐ mild ☐ moderate ☐ severe ☐ medial ☐ lateral	**Joint line pain:** ☐ none ☐ mild ☐ moderate ☐ severe ☐ medial ☐ lateral
Patella tracking: ☐ normal ☐ medial ☐ lateral	**Patella tracking:** ☐ normal ☐ medial ☐ lateral

(with kind permission from Genzyme Biosurgery)

CARTICEL℠ Service Registry

Registry Number: _____
Implantation Number: _____

Patient Initials ☐ ☐ ☐

TO BE COMPLETED BY CLINICAL STAFF

Indicate month of follow-up or subsequent visit number
☐ 6 ☐ 12 ☐ 24 ☐ S1 ☐ S2 ☐ S3

3/12/96

Clinician's Evaluation

Date of evaluation:
☐ ☐ ☐ ☐ ☐ ☐

Rate the patient according to the following scale.

☐ 1 ☐ 2 ☐ 3 ☐ 4 ☐ 5 ☐ 6 ☐ 7 ☐ 8 ☐ 9 ☐ 10
    poor   fair   good   very good   excellent

Poor (2) .... Patient has significant limitations in daily activities.

Fair (4) .... Patient has moderate limitations that affect daily activities, no sports possible.

Good (6) .... Patient has some limitations with sports but can participate by compensating.

Very good (8) ... Patient has only a few limitations with sports.

Excellent (10) .. Patient is able to do whatever they wish (any sport) with no problems.

Knee Examination

Conduct knee exam on both knees.

LEFT KNEE		RIGHT KNEE	
Extension:	**Flexion:**	**Extension:**	**Flexion:**
☐☐☐ °	☐☐☐ °	☐☐☐ °	☐☐☐ °

Alignment: (LEFT KNEE)
☐ extreme varus < 0°
☐ varus 0° to < 5°
☐ normal 5° to < 10°
☐ valgus 10° to < 15°
☐ extreme valgus ≥ 15°

Alignment: (RIGHT KNEE)
☐ extreme varus < 0°
☐ varus 0° to < 5°
☐ normal 5° to < 10°
☐ valgus 10° to < 15°
☐ extreme valgus ≥ 15°

Anteroposterior stability (mm): (LEFT KNEE)
☐ < 5
☐ 5 to < 10
☐ ≥ 10

Anteroposterior stability (mm): (RIGHT KNEE)
☐ < 5
☐ 5 to < 10
☐ ≥ 10

Mediolateral stability: (LEFT KNEE)
☐ < 5°
☐ 5° to < 10°
☐ 10° to < 15°
☐ ≥ 15°

Mediolateral stability: (RIGHT KNEE)
☐ < 5°
☐ 5° to < 10°
☐ 10° to < 15°
☐ ≥ 15°

Knee Examination (cont.)

LEFT KNEE	RIGHT KNEE

Crepitus: (LEFT)
☐ none
☐ mild
☐ moderate
☐ severe

Crepitus: (RIGHT)
☐ none
☐ mild
☐ moderate
☐ severe

Effusion: (LEFT)
☐ none
☐ mild
☐ moderate
☐ severe

Effusion: (RIGHT)
☐ none
☐ mild
☐ moderate
☐ severe

Joint line pain: (LEFT)
☐ none
☐ mild
☐ moderate
☐ severe
☐ medial   ☐ lateral

Joint line pain: (RIGHT)
☐ none
☐ mild
☐ moderate
☐ severe
☐ medial   ☐ lateral

Patella tracking: (LEFT)
☐ normal
☐ medial
☐ lateral

Patella tracking: (RIGHT)
☐ normal
☐ medial
☐ lateral

Rehabilitation

Current type of rehabilitation:
☐ prescribed rehabilitation
☐ at home exercise program

Rehabilitation program:
☐ ahead of schedule
☐ on schedule
☐ behind schedule

In the case of an adverse event:
1. Call Genzyme Medical Affairs Europe at +31-35-6991299.
2. Complete an Adverse Event Page.
3. Fax completed Adverse Event Page to Genzyme Medical Affairs Europe, Hans Ebels, MD at +31-35-6948756.

Lysholm Score

Limp (5 points)

None	5
Slight or periodical	3
Severe and constant	0

Support (5 points)

Full support	5
Stick or crutch	3
Weight bearing impossible	0

Stairclimbing (10 points)

No problems	10
Slightly impaired	6
One step at a time	2
Unable	0

Squatting (5 points)

No problems	5
Slightly impaired	4
Not past 90°	2
Unable	0

Walking, running and jumping (70 points)

A. Instability

Never giving way	30
Rarely during athletic or other severe exertion	25
Frequently during athletic or other severe exertion (or unable to participate)	20
Occasionally in daily activities	10
Often in daily activities	5
Every step	0

B. Pain

None	30
Inconstant and slight during severe exertion	25
Marked on giving way	20
Marked during severe exertion	15
Marked on or after walking more than 2 km	10
Marked on or after walking less than 2 km	5
Constant and severe	0

C. Swelling

None	10
With giving way	7
On severe excertion	5
On ordinary excertion	2
Constant	0

Atrophy of thigh (5 points)

None	5
1–2 cm	3
More than 2 cm	0

Tegner Activity Score

10. Competitive sports
Soccer – national and international elite

9. Competitive sports
Soccer – lower divisions
Ice hockey
Wrestling
Gymnastics

8. Competitive sports
Bandy
Squash or Badminton
Athletics (jumping etc.)
Downhill skiing

7. Competitive sports
Tennis
Athletics (running)
Motorcross, speedway
Handball
Basketball
Recreational sports
Soccer
Bandy and ice hockey
Squash
Athletics (jumping)
Cross-country track findings

6. Recreational sports
Tennis and badminton
Handball
Basketball
Downhill skiing
Jogging, at least five times a week

5. Work
Heavy labor
Competitive sports
Cycling
Cross-country skiing
Recreational sports
Jogging on uneven ground at least twice weekly

4. Work
Moderately heavy labor
Recreational sports
Cycling
Cross-country skiing
Jogging on even ground at least twice a weekly

3. Work
Light labor
Competitive and recreational sports
Swimming
Walking in forest possible

2. Work
Light labor
Walking on uneven ground possible but impossible to walk in forest

1. Work
Sedentary work
Walking on even ground possible

0. Sick leave or disability pension because of knee problems

Freiburg Ankle Score (FAS)

Untersuchungsbogen Sprunggelenk

Orthopädische Klinik
Albert-Ludwigs-Universität
Freiburg

rechts (1) / links (2)..................... ____

Trauma ja (1) / nein (2)............... ____

Beruf...

Schmerz .... ____

kein Schmerz 30
gelegentlicher Schmerz unter Belastung (Sport) -
keine Beeinträchtigung des täglichen Lebens
.... 25
leichter Schmerz unter Belastung (Sport) geringe
Beeinträchtigung des täglichen Lebens 20
starker Schmerz unter Belastung - Sport nicht
möglich - deutliche Beeinträchtigung des täglichen
Lebens - gelegentlicher Schmerz auch in Ruhe -
Schmerzmittel bei Bedarf 15
ständiger Schmerz - regelmäßig Schmerzmittel
.... 10

Stabilität/Unsicherheit beim Gehen bzw. Laufen .... ____

keine Unsicherheit..................................... 10
leichte Unsicherheit beim Laufen bzw. Gehen auf
unebenem Untergrund 8
Unsicherheit beim Gehen auf
ebenem Boden.. 6
Gehen nur mit Schiene/ orthopädischem Schuh
möglich.. 0

Leistungsfähigkeit/schmerzfreie Gehstrecke (Limitierung wegen Sprunggelenk)........................... ____

unbegrenzte Gehstrecke /
Belastungsdauer 10
Belastungsdauer kleiner als 1 Stunde........ 6
nur wenige Schritte/in der Wohnung/mit Gehhilfe
.... 0

Patienten Daten

Name: ....
Vorname: ....
Geburtsdatum: ....
Strasse:..
PLZ: ....
Ort: ....
Tel: ....
Fax:...

Gang...____

flüssig, kein Hinken 10
flüssig, leichtes Hinken................................ 8
schwerfällig, deutliches Hinken 6
Stock/Unterarmgehstützen........................... 0

Umfangsdifferenz verletzt/gesund (über Außenknöchel) ....____

0 cm 10
0-2 cm 6
>2 cm 0

Beweglichkeit

Dorsalextension......................____

30°.. 10
20°.. 8
10°.. 6
nicht möglich 0

Plantarflexion........................____

40°.. 10
30°.. 8
20°.. 6
10°.. 4
nicht möglich 0

Kraft/Stabilität ....____

Zehenstand möglich: 10 Wiederholungen . 10
Zehenstand möglich: 5 Wiederholungen..... 8
Zehenstand möglich: 1 Wiederholung........ 6
Zehenstand nicht möglich 0

SCORE TOTAL ....____/100

Important Analytic Methods

Histology

Histological analysis is used to specifically stain characteristic structures of a histological section in order to identify them. Coloured tissue morphology may then be evaluated, described and analyzed microscopically.

"Classic" stainings may be used in both unfixed sections (fresh or frozen sections) and in formalin fixed, paraffin embedded sections. For the identification of enzymes or metabolic products unfixed cryosections are preferred.

Hematoxylin-Eosin (HE) according to Ehrlich

In HE stainings all basophilic cell and tissue structures such as nucleus chromatin, some cytoplasm components and parts of cartilage matrix appear blue-violet. Acidophilic components such as cell cytoplasm, intercellular substances, muscle tissue and fibrous tissue appear red. HE is the most commonly used nucleus stain (see Fig. 1).

Safranin-O

Safranin-O (Saf-O) stains nuclei black, cytoplasm grey-green, intact cartilage matrix as well as mucines and mast cell granules orange or red (Fig. 62).

Hematoxylin-van Gieson

Hematoxylin-van Gieson stains nuclei dark brown or black, muscle tissue and elastic connective tissue yellow-brown and mature collagenous and reticular connective tissue intensively red. This method is used to identify the content of fibrous tissue in fibrosis or sclerosis. Immature collagen or collagen precursors cannot be stained with this method.

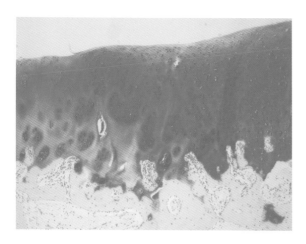

Fig. 62. Histological section of intact, ovine articular cartilage, Safranin-O staining.

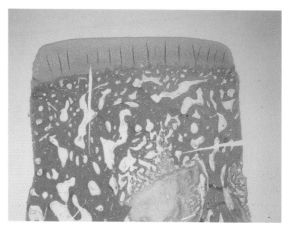

Fig. 63. Histological section of intact, ovine articular cartilage, Hematoxylin-van Gieson staining.

Counterstaining with Elastica-van Gieson stains elastic fibres black and therefore allows differentiation between different connective tissues.

Alcian blue

Alcian blue staining is specifically used to identify acidic mucopolysaccharides. They appear bright red, nuclei light red with a light violet background. Differentiation between sulfate- and carboxyl-groups is not possible (Fig. 64).

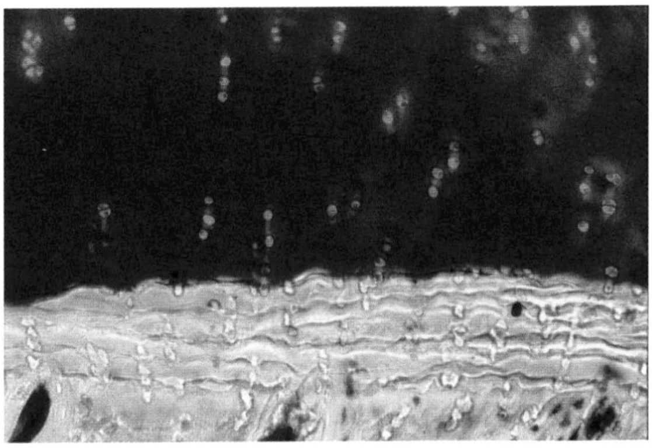

Fig. 64. Histological section of regenerating, equine articular cartilage following ACT, Alcian-blue staining (with kind permission of M. Sittinger and C. Kaps, Berlin, Germany).

Alcian blue-PAS

Alcian blue-PAS stains both acidic and neutral mucopolysaccharides. PAS-negative acidic mucous substances appear bright blue, neutral mucous substances and polysaccharides red. PAS-positive, acidic mucous substances appear in a combination of these colours.

Toluidine blue

Toluidine blue may be used to determine viability of chondrocytes (Fig. 65).

Immunohistochemistry

Immunohistochemical methods are used to identify certain proteins in or on cells as well as in tissues.

Immunohistochemical methods detect certain proteins (precisely speaking: epitopes) as antigens using specifically produced antibodies. These are then made visible using secondary, fluorescent antibodies which bond to primary antibodies. Antibody-epitope complexes may then be evaluated using fluorescence microscopy (Figs. 66, 67).

Fig. 65. Histological section of intact human articular cartilage, Toluidine-blue staining (with kind permission of S. Roberts, Oswestry, UK).

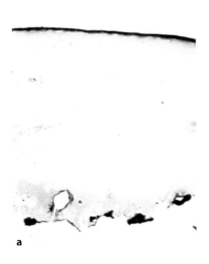

a

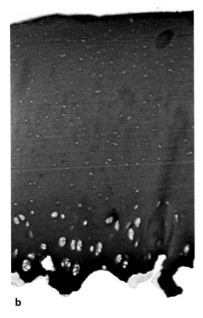

b

Fig. 66 a, b. Intact human articular cartilage. Immunohisto-chemical identification of collagen type I (**a**) and type II (**b**) (with kind permission of S. Roberts, Oswestry, UK).

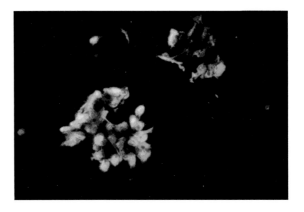

Fig. 67. Immunofluorescence on a cryosection, identifying hyaluronan synthase 3 (HAS3, green) on ovine chondrocytes in 3D-hydrogel culture after 10 weeks (in collaboration with H. Kurz, E. Mrosek and J. Schagemann, Freiburg, Germany).

Polymerase chain reaction (PCR)

PCR is a method derived from molecular biology. It allows amplification of specific DNA fragments. Certain DNA-sequences can be synthesized using DNA-polymerases. Two synthetic oligonucleotides (so-called primers) build a frame around the DNA-sequence of interest. By means of exponential accumulation small DNA samples (10^{-9}–10^{-15} g) may be identified or used for genetic purposes after multifold repetition of the procedure.

RNA has to be translated into DNA by using RNA-dependent DNA-polymerases for the detection of RNA-sequences.

Subject Index